ISBN-13: 978-1519108944

Copyright © 2013 by R.O.S. Therapy Systems, L.L.C.
All rights reserved including the right of reproduction in whole or in part.

Published by:
R.O.S. Therapy Systems, L.L.C.
Greensboro, NC
888-352-9788
www.ROSTherapySystems.com

Activities 101 Complete
Table of Contents

I)	The People We Serve	3
II)	Communicating and Motivating for Success	39
III)	What is "Activities"?	72
IV)	Importance of Family Involvement in Engaging Activities	84
V)	How to Engage Clients	96
VI)	When Should Activities Be Conducted with Clients?	119
VII)	Sample Activities	134
VIII)	Resources	154

Section I

The People We Serve

Introduction to Aging

While aging is often associated with declining health, current research suggests there are some things people can do to remain healthier longer. For instance, maintaining a positive attitude has been shown to correlate with better health among the elderly. Older individuals with more positive attitudes and emotions engage in less risky behavior and have lower stress levels, both of which are correlated with better overall health.

To best comprehend the aging process, one should become familiar with the terminology and some of the disease processes used when discussing the aging process or the elderly.

When we think of aging, we often think of the physical aspects, or the outward signs, that indicate the aging process has begun such as graying hair, less skin elasticity (wrinkles), and a slower gait (more unsteady on our feet). In normal aging, three processes take place: the physical changes, the psychological factors (e.g., the mind, a person's feelings, and overall mental health), and the social changes (changes within family dynamics and relationships).

Responsibilities, relationships, and roles change with age. Psychosocial changes include the ability to change or adapt. Some people cope better with the aging process depending on their attitudes, finances, health, support systems, and spiritual beliefs. No two people age in the same manner. Acceptance, adjustment, and adaptation are all uniquely personal.

Physical Changes with Aging

The Integumentary System (Skin)

As a person ages, their skin becomes dry, has less elasticity, develops wrinkles, and is increasingly prone to bruising and tearing. In addition, sweat glands decrease and produce less oil. Age spots start appearing, especially in areas exposed to sunlight. Though wrinkles become increasingly pronounced during this time, most lines in the face form early in life (generally in the mid-twenties), and are associated with common and repetitive facial expressions. It is said that smoking can accelerate the aging process. However, whether or not someone has smoked during their life, water and lotion can aid the skin by adding moisture.

Physical Changes seen with aging –

- Wrinkling of the skin
- Loss of hair color
- Thickening of the nails
- Weakening of the blood vessels (causing spider veins also known as varicose veins)
- Diminished sweat gland production
- More visible moles and darkening of the skin (age spots)
- Potential teeth problems (loosening, dentures)

The Sensory System (Hearing, Touch, Smell, Taste, and Sight)

The sensory system is not typically considered a true body "system," yet some components of the sensory system that aid a person in moving through life such as hearing, sight, taste, smell, and touch do change with the aging process. The eyes have a decreased tolerance for glare, an increased sensitivity to light (when lights are turned on after being in a dark room), and a person's peripheral vision is decreased. Decreased hearing can result from thickening of the ear canal or an increase of wax build-up in the ear. During the aging process, the ability to distinguish between taste and smell also changes to a different extent for each person. The sense of touch can be more diminished due to thickening of the skin in some parts of the body such as the fingertips and palms, yet it can be more sensitive in other areas due to thinning.

Sensory issues typically seen with aging –

- Cataracts (murkiness or film that forms over the eye, usually do to protein changes)
- Glaucoma (build-up of pressure in the eye, generally leads to blindness)
- Tinnitus (ringing or buzzing in the ears)
- Slower to react to sense of touch
- Need stronger odors to recognize/distinguish smells
- Imbalance due to changes in the ears and equilibrium issues
- Intolerance for bright lights and glare

The Cardiovascular System (Heart, Veins, and Blood)

The heart tends to enlarge with age, while the heart's ability to contract decreases. Plaque can build up on the inside of the blood vessels, which makes them more rigid. The heart's left ventricle thickens and the aorta dilates. Heart valves become more rigid and thicken, and arteries can become less efficient. Fatty foods, lack of regular exercise, and some hereditary issues can lend to other increased issues with aging.

The major types of heart disease are Coronary Heart Disease, Cardiomyopathy, Cardiovascular Disease, Ischemic Heart Disease, Congestive Heart Failure, Inflammatory Heart Disease, Valvular Heart Disease, and Hypertensive Heart Disease (though even more specific subtypes exist in the International Classification of Disease code).

Coronary Artery Disease is a disorder of the arteries caused by the accumulation of atheromatous plaques within the walls of the arteries that supply the myocardium (heart muscle). The build-up of these plaques can lead to an occlusion, or blockage, of the blood supply to the heart, thus leading to ischemia (lack of blood supply) and damage or death to the heart muscle tissue (myocardium). This disorder leads to symptoms of chest pain (most commonly in the left arm or neck), difficulty breathing, sweating, a sense of impending doom, and vomiting. The heart is weakened by the release of lactic acid leading to lower functioning in all organs, particularly the brain, kidneys, and lungs because these organs require the most blood flow.

Cardiomyopathy literally means "heart muscle disease" (myo = muscle, pathy = disease). It is the deterioration of the function of the myocardium (i.e., the actual heart muscle) for any reason. People with cardiomyopathy are often at risk for arrhythmia and sudden cardiac death.

Valvular Heart Disease refers to problems with the functioning of the valves of the heart (the aortic and mitral valves on the left side or the pulmonary and tricuspid valves on the right side). Valve problems may be congenital (inborn) or acquired (due to another cause later in life). Treatment may be with medication but, depending on the severity, often involves valve repair or replacement (insertion of an artificial heart valve from either a pig or a metal valve).

Inflammatory Heart Disease, or swelling of the heart, can lead to inefficient closing of the heart valves, which reduces the efficiency of each pump of the heart. The causes of inflammatory heart disease are both extrinsic (caused by factors outside the myocardium) and intrinsic (weakness in the heart muscle without obvious external reason).

Ischemia is the most common cause of a cardiomyopathy, along with other triggers such as alcoholic cardiomyopathy, nutritional diseases affecting the heart, and hypertensive cardiomyopathy.

Intrinsic Cardiomyopathies can be Dilated Cardiomyopathy (left ventricle is enlarged and the pumping function is diminished), Hypertrophic Cardiomyopathy (heart muscle is thickened due to gene mutations encoding sarcomeric proteins), Arhythmogenic Right Ventricular Cardiomyopathy (electrical disturbance of the heart in which heart muscle is replaced by fibrous scar tissue), and Restrictive Cardiomyopathy (ventricle walls are stiff, but may not be thickened, and resist the normal filling of the heart with blood).

Since 1950, the prevalence of heart disease has been slowly declining because many of the risk factors have been identified and can be controlled with modified diet and attention to health behaviors such as smoking and exercise. Furthermore, evidence proves that although early intervention is helpful, it is never too late to change one's life and reduce exposure to risk factors. Having two or more risk factors dramatically boosts one's chance of developing coronary atherosclerosis, because detrimental effects of each risk factor are multiplied by the effects of the others. Having high cholesterol also adds to the risk of this disease.

The following factors provide the highest level of risk: smoking, high blood pressure, high blood LDL (low density lipoproteins), diabetes mellitus, family history, advancing age, high blood homocysteine, physical inactivity, obesity, stress, menopause, being male, certain personality characteristics, and high blood iron levels. The actual amount of increase in risk from each one depends on when the risk factor existed; its intensity, frequency, and duration; and its interaction with other risk factors.

There is an age-related increase in the release of norepinephrine, a stress hormone. The concentration of norepinephrine reaches higher levels at older ages, thereby providing increased stimulation to the heart and leading to a greater risk of oxidative damage. With age, there is also an increase in the amount of blood remaining in the left ventricle after contraction. This leads to an inhibition of blood flow from the lungs as well as more blood in the lungs, known as pulmonary congestion. The older heart consumes more oxygen to pump the same amount of blood.

Heart issues typically seen with aging –
- Angina (pain that occurs when the heart doesn't receive enough oxygenated blood)
- Arteriosclerosis (arteries harden – related to smoking, obesity, poor diet or genetics)
- Congestive Heart Failure (CHF) – heart loses ability to pump blood and oxygen to other parts of the body
- Coronary Artery Disease (clots or fatty deposits around the heart)
- Hypertension (high blood pressure)
- Phlebitis (inflammation of veins in the legs)
- Transient Ischemic Attack (TIA) – mini-stroke

The Respiratory System (Mouth, Nose, Sinuses, Lungs, etc.)

The lungs' ability to expand and contract decreases with age. In turn, the ability for efficient air exchange changes with aging. The diaphragm and the thorax also weaken with age. The effectiveness of coughing and the ability to cough up mucus also decreases. The blood flow to organs decreases, which can decrease the amount of oxygen to the various organs and cause lung damage. Oftentimes, deep breathing and exercise can assist with this aging process.

Breathing issues typically seen with aging –

- COPD (Chronic Obstructive Pulmonary Disease) – bronchitis and emphysema, difficulty breathing

- Emphysema – chronic condition when lungs are unable to properly contract and expand, lends to poor oxygen quality

- Bronchitis (inflammation of the bronchi) – causes a repetitive cough and excessive mucus. Some people can contract this several times a year (chronic).

- Pneumonia (lung inflammation) – typically caused by a virus or bacteria and can often lead to death in an older person if not promptly and properly treated

- Lung Cancer – often caused by exposure to hazardous materials or smoking and other products inhaled in the lungs

The Musculoskeletal System (Bones, Muscles, Joints, Ligaments, Cartilage, and Tendons)

Bones become thinner and more brittle with aging. The loss of bone in the spine, or thinning of the disks in between the vertebrae, causes people to lose a few inches or become shorter after the age of 30. 206 bones and numerous joints allow movement in the body. Exercise and consuming calcium can assist with the strengthening of bones. Joints also become more rigid as the cartilage in joints decreases. Exercise is recommended to assist with this process. The body contains more than 500 muscles which can start losing their mass after about age 30 and decreases more rapidly after midlife. Reaction time is slower with aging, and the ability to exert muscle strength also decreases. Exercise can assist with maintaining good muscle tone and slow the process of muscle turning to fat. Women tend to gain more weight around their mid-section as they age, almost at a 2 to 1 rate more than men.

Many seniors also suffer from arthritis, or inflammation of the joints; it is officially the leading cause of disability among Americans. There are more than 100 known rheumatic diseases characterized by problems in and around the joints. Estimates of those affected vary. Among older adults, about 65% report some type of arthritis. However, doctors report about 33% of older adults with arthritis. The Arthritis Foundation estimates 66 million people with doctor-diagnosed arthritis. Therefore, about 1 in 5 people in America have problems with arthritis.

Arthritis is more of an issue for women than men – partly because they live longer and partly because of gender differences in the relative size of supportive muscles.

Various exercises have been developed to alleviate some of the issues associated with arthritis. Certain exercises have been shown to help develop a better sleep pattern, help with weight control, maintain heart health, increase bone and muscle strength, and decrease depression and fatigue. Moving joints daily helps keep them fully mobile and strengthens the surrounding muscles that support the joints. Also, joint movement transports nutrients and waste products to and from the cartilage, the material which protects and cushions the ends of the bones.

Rheumatoid arthritis can cause inflammation of the tissue around the joints as well as other organs of the body. As an autoimmune disease, the joints and neighboring tissues are attacked by the body's immune system, causing inflammation and affecting other organs and tissues in the body. Chronic inflammation causes deformities and leads to the destruction of the cartilage, bone, and ligaments. The pain a person feels is not necessarily related to the actual damage. One can have pain, stiffness, and swelling with either limited damage or extended damage and fewer symptoms.

Bone issues typically seen with aging –

- Osteoporosis – weakening of the bones, which can cause fractures – typically a broken hip, which causes a fall

- Rheumatoid arthritis (inflammation of connective tissue) – causes stiffness and joint pain, usually chronic

- Osteoarthritis (degenerative joint disease) – another form of arthritis caused by loss of cartilage, which exposes bones to pain

- Osteoporosis (a bone disease) – bone tissue is absorbed at a faster rate than new bones or bone tissue can be formed, resulting in a reduction of bone mass which can cause fractures

The Gastrointestinal System (Digestive System)

The digestive system includes the process when food enters your mouth until it is eliminated. Digestion involves many organs and other parts of the body. Teeth are more brittle and the enamel tends to be thinner with the older person, yet the fact that many older people wear dentures is a result of lack of preventative methods and available technology. When a person ages, their mouth is drier as the mucus glands dry and saliva is decreased. Taste buds are reduced as well as gastric acids and enzymes. The stomach takes longer to empty into the intestines when a person is older and the liver gets smaller and has less capacity. The intestinal muscles also become slower. (This reflects the thicker middle section on aging clients after midlife). As the digestive process ages, what a person eats and their ability to chew and swallow can be greatly affected. This change in diet and ability to process foods could cause discomfort including gas, loose stools, and other digestive ailments. The loss of muscle strength can also have adverse effects on elimination, causing accidents in older age as the muscles around the organs weaken and react slower.

Digestive issues typically seen with aging –

- Diverticulosis – a weakening of the intestinal walls in which sacs/pouches protrude and become infected

- Periodontal disease – inflammation of tissue surrounding the teeth and gums tend to recede from repeated brushing and simple wear and tear

- Hiatal hernias – part of the stomach is pushed through the diaphragm

- Cirrhosis – inflammation in the liver usually caused by poor nutrition or continued consumption of large amounts of alcohol

- Glycogen – energy storage diminished

- Intramuscular fat increases

The Urinary System (Kidneys, Urethra and Bladder)

Bladder muscles become weaker with aging and bladder capacity decreases as well. Older people experience more urgency and involuntary loss of urine. Sometimes even laughing, coughing or sneezing can cause pressure on the muscles, which can cause accidents. This stress incontinence can cause people to alter their lifestyle by staying closer to the bathroom or not engaging in their favorite activities for fear of having an accident.

Urinary issues typically seen with aging –

- Incontinence – inability to control bladder or bowel functions due to physical or cognitive changes with aging

- UTI (urinary tract infection) – infection of the bladder, kidney or other part of the urinary tract caused by bacteria

- Renal failure – inability of the kidneys to perform normally as we age

The Reproductive System

During menopause, the aging factors related to the reproductive system include a decrease in sexual response, weakening of the pelvic muscles, and a reduction in estrogen levels for women. The cervix and uterus decrease in size, the fallopian tubes atrophy (dry up/shrink), and estrogen and ovulation production ceases. During andropause, male testes decrease in size, and it takes longer for a male to have an erection. Older adults are able to engage in satisfying sexual activity with the assistance of lubricants and an understanding sexual partner. The myth that older people have a decreased interest or desire for sexual activity is inaccurate. It is generally the opposite, as many couples find retirement age a more freeing time to engage in a meaningful relationship without the interference of children, jobs, and other responsibilities. In many long-term care facilities, there may be a lack of opportunity or privacy, but not necessarily a lack of interest or ability.

Sexual issues typically seen with aging –

Males –

- Delayed ejaculation
- Slower sexual response
- Decreased sperm count (yet still enough for reproduction)
- Decreased testosterone levels

Females –

- Thinning tissue of the vaginal wall
- Decreased estrogen levels
- Weakening of breast muscles/tissues
- Decreased vaginal lubrication

The Endocrine System

The endocrine system is comprised of glands that release hormones into the blood stream on a specific basis to control and help operate bodily functions. In addition to the two reproductive glands mentioned in the reproductive system, the endocrine system also includes the pituitary and pineal body (located near the brain), the thyroid (located in the throat area), and the adrenal and pancreas (located near the stomach). The pituitary gland, located under the brain, works with the hypothalamus to control the production of urine, the growth process, and the work of many other glands. Since the pituitary gland has so much influence throughout the body, it is sometimes called the 'master' gland. The adrenal glands, located on top of the kidneys, release adrenaline and cortisone, which controls the water to salt balance and proteins in the body. The thyroid glands regulate the cells and metabolism in the body. The pancreas controls the digestive system, discussed earlier in this document.

Endocrine issues typically seen with aging –

- Decrease in levels of estrogen and progesterone
- Decreased insulin production

- Increased levels of parathormone/thyroid stimulating hormones
- Hormone secretions decrease
- Glands become less active or decrease in size, which causes a decrease in production of hormones
- Addison's Disease – a deficiency of hormones that causes weak muscles and fatigue
- Diabetes – the body's inability to produce the necessary insulin to control sugar levels
- Grave's Disease – hyperthyroidism caused by an increase in the production of the thyroid hormone, which causes weight loss, fatigue, and an enlarged thyroid (hypothyroidism is a decrease in thyroid hormone production)
- Cushing's Syndrome – the body produces large amounts of adrenal cortex hormones

The Immune System

In conjunction with the thalamus gland mentioned above, the immune system starts to decline around age 30 and continues to decline. As a result, older adults are more susceptible to infections and illnesses. White blood cells, which fight infections, are less effective than they once were in younger age. Vaccinations, routine physician visits, and avoiding overexposure to illness combined with proper diet and exercise can help control the susceptibility of the immune system.

Immune System issues typically seen with aging –

- Decreased white blood cell production
- Viruses and other infections become more life threatening

The Nervous System (Brain, Nerves, and Spinal Cord)

Key functions of this system include coordinating and operating all bodily functions. The weight of the brain decreases with age, and the neurons also decrease in numbers. The central nervous system (CNS) includes the brain, spinal cord, and the membranes that surround it. The cerebellum is responsible for muscle functions. The cerebrum, the biggest part of the brain, is responsible for thinking, reasoning, and voluntary movements. The brain stem, which contains the neurons, controls involuntary movements in the major organs in the body. Normal functioning such as memory, language, comprehension, judgment, abstract thinking, and orientation change during a disease process involving the nervous system.

Nervous System issues typically seen with aging –

- Loss of neurons

- Decreased tactile (touch) sensitivity – see skin system

- Memory changes – due to a disease process (not normal memory changes associated with healthy aging)

- Decreased reaction time

- Cerebrovascular accident (CVA) – blood supply to the brain is cut off, which can hamper speech, vision, and memory as well as weakening of the muscles

- Multi-infarct dementia – caused by strokes and can be the result of a build-up, or plaque, in the brain (Dementia is triggered by a different disease process such as hypertension or heart disease.)

- Multiple Sclerosis (MS) – this disease develops slowly and results from problems in the brain and spinal cord that control motor and sensory skills

- Parkinson's disease – a progressive disease that involves shaking, very slow movements as a result of rigid muscles, and a chemical imbalance in the brain which alters the brain's ability to transmit information

Functional disorders may include –

- Agnosia – inability to perceive an object or a person in a normal fashion

- Amnesia – memory loss which could be permanent

- Apraxia – a decline in fine or gross motor skills, as a result of inability to perform previously learned functions

- Aphasia – loss of language and understanding as well as impaired communication

Dementia

According to the National Institutes of Health, dementia is "a clinical state with many different causes, characterized by a decline from a previously attained intellectual level." *Merriam-Webster's Dictionary* defines dementia as "a usually progressive condition (as Alzheimer's disease) marked by deteriorated cognitive functioning often with emotional apathy." Dementia is one of the most commonly seen conditions in long-term care facilities and nursing homes. This disease process requires specialized training and programming.

The cause of dementia is a brain dysfunction which disrupts both the thought process and perception. The onset of dementia is generally slow with small, subtle problems noted in normal daily life including restlessness and forgetfulness. Once the disease progresses, the problems become more noticeable such as unfamiliarity of family members and friends and an increase in disruptive or unsocial behaviors. The sensory or motor skills of a person can also become increasing altered or disrupted.

There are two main types of dementia: reversible and irreversible. Reversible dementia is brought on by a disease or a condition such as infection, intoxication, depression, a reaction to medication(s), heart or lung problems, and other disorders that may deprive the brain of oxygen. Irreversible dementia is characterized by a pathological disease that is progressive with no other cause identified. The most common form of irreversible dementia is Alzheimer's disease.

Alzheimer's Disease

This disease is the primary dementia in the elderly today. While the cause is still unknown, the disease is marked by a slow deterioration of cognitive function until death. Alzheimer's disease was named after Dr. Alois Alzheimer in 1907. It is estimated that more than 5 million individuals over the age of 65 have been diagnosed with this disease in the United States alone. Currently, no cure for Alzheimer's disease exists. The deterioration of this disease varies from person to person. Thought, language, and memory are affected in specific portions of the brain marked by twisted plaque materials – dead and dying cells. Alzheimer's can often be initially mistaken for senile dementia, yet the symptoms become more noticeable over time with increasingly impaired memory loss and difficulty in planning and other thought processes. The ability to perform daily activities (i.e., bathing, dressing, etc.) declines at a more rapid pace until the individual can no longer provide self-care and requires full or assisted care.

The Alzheimer's Association provides the following as a guide to possible changes in function and loss of abilities.

1. Memory impairment

    a) Inability to remember important information (an event, meeting, trip, child or grandchild) – more than occasional forgetfulness

    b) Inability to remember/recall well-learned information and/or inability to learn new information (how to operate a familiar machine – using a telephone)

    c) Perseveration – repetitive movements or persistence in statements or questions (tapping, folding, hand-wringing or saying a phrase over and over)

2. Disorientation to time

    a) Dressing inappropriately for the season or the weather (heavy coat in summer)

    b) Missing important appointments or deadlines

3. Disorientation to place

    a) Getting lost in familiar surroundings (losing the way home from the workplace which has been the same for many years, possible unexplained absences where person has difficulty finding directions from one place to another)

    b) Inability to orient in an unfamiliar place (finding the bathroom)

4. Impairment of judgment

    a) A change in decision-making ability (poor household decisions or business/financial decisions)

    b) Difficulty concentrating

    c) Inappropriate judgment (calling police for unwarranted suspicions)

    d) Inappropriate control of impulses (exhibitionism, sexually inappropriate remarks, actions, change in toileting habits such as urinating on street, marked change in buying or saving habits)

5. Language impairment

    a) Change in ability to communicate effectively

    b) Marked change in vocabulary (soft-spoken words to harsh profanity)

    c) Change in language skills (frequent searching for words, particularly nouns)

    d) Conversations which are incomprehensible or irrelevant, losses in train of thought

    e) Difficulty understanding what is said, may become argumentative or combative

    f) Tendency to repeat the same words or phrases

6. Decline in capabilities and routine, daily activities

   a) Change in eating or dietary habits (dramatic change in preference for sweets, salty foods or condiments)

   b) Change in sleep patterns

   c) Significant change in the way a person dresses or grooms (not bathing)

   d) Regressive change in table manners (using fingers or eating directly from serving bowls)

   e) Marked change in reading habits (not reading the newspaper)

   f) Marked change in writing abilities (the mechanics of writing evidenced in checkbook from one year to another – name not signed in designated area)

   g) Change in ability to perform simple perceptual tasks (unlock door or familiar tasks such as paying bills, evidenced in nonpayment or duplicate payment of bills which were usually paid on time)

   h) Loss of measured intellectual ability (evidenced from former records, school, military, employment, testing, films, artwork or written material)

   i) Marked change or difference in interests and activities

7. Change in personality and/or marked difficulty maintaining social function

   a) Noticeable personality change (confident to indecisive, extroverted to withdrawn, accommodating to demanding or vice versa)

   b) Difficulty in maintaining friends and former social relationships

   c) Increased dependency

8. Changes in expression of feelings

   a) Withdrawal or disassociation from activities and/or situations

   b) Inappropriate or unwarranted anger, frequent crying in one who never or rarely cried

   c) Dramatic mood swings from happy to sad, stubborn to docile or vice versa

9. Thinking disturbances

    a) Unwarranted suspiciousness (thinking food is poisoned or that people are stealing things)

    b) Seeing/hearing/touching things and/or people that are not there, imaginary friends or enemies (in mirror or on TV)

    c) Imaginary powers such as invincibleness

10. Job performance

    a) Marked change in vocational interest

    b) Missed deadlines or appointments

    c) Reduced efficiency on the job

    d) Catastrophic reactions to problem situations

11. Other influences

    a) Marked change in acceptance of physical limitations

    b) Drug or alcohol abuse

    c) Marked change because of other illness

Knowing and understanding how a dementia diagnosis is made and how the different stages in each disease progress is most important in planning meaningful programs for clients with dementia. Evaluations for a diagnosis can include the following tests:

- A full medical exam
- An EEG, EKG, MRI, and other tests
- A full blood profile
- An assessment of social issues and lifestyle factors
- Cognitive test results

One of the most common tools for diagnosing dementia is called the Mini Mental State Examination (MMSE) created by Folstein and McHugh in 1975. The exam is administered by a clinician and includes questions involving the date, state, month, and country; recall questions, testing language, sentence construction, and ability. The scores from the eleven questions are tallied, then utilized to determine the level of individual impairment. One version of the test is shown below. Its use is starting to fade because it doesn't catch many early-stage patients and can result in a fair amount of false positives.

Maximum Score	Score	
		ORIENTATION
5	( )	What is the: (year) (season) (date) (day) (month)
5	( )	Where are we: (state) (county) (town) (facility) (floor)
		REGISTRATION
3	( )	Name three objects and have person repeat them back. Give one point for each correct answer on the first trial. 1._____ 2._____ 3._____ Then repeat them (up to 6x) until all three are learned. [Number of trials ____]
		ATTENTION AND CALCULATION
5	( )	Serial 7's. Count backwards from 100 by serial 7's. One point for each correct answer. Stop after 5 answers. [93 86 79 72 65] Alternatively spell "world" backwards. [D - L - R - O - W]
		RECALL
3	( )	Ask fo rthe names of the three objects learned above. Give one point for each correct answer.
		LANGUAGE
9	( )	Name: a pen (1 point) and a watch (1 point) Repeat the following: "No ifs, ands, or buts" (1 point) Follow a three-stage command: "Take this paper in your [non-dominant] hand, fold it in half and put it on the floor". (3 points) [1 point for each part correctly performed] Read to self and then do: "Close your eyes" (1 point) Write a sentence [subject, verb and makes sense] (1 point) Copy design [5 sided geometric figure; 2 points must intersect] (1 point)

Score: ___/30   Alert   Overtly Anxious   Concentration Difficulty   Drowsy

CLOSE YOUR EYES

Another diagnostic method utilized to determine cognitive impairment is the Global Deterioration Scale developed by Reisburg, Ferris, Crook and DeLeon in 1982. With this method, individuals are categorized into seven different stages:

Stage 1 – (No cognitive decline) no memory complaints and no evidence of problems during the exam

Stage 2 – (Very mild cognitive decline) forgetfulness of names and familiar objects

Stage 3 – (Mild cognitive decline) performance declines, concentration problems, some denial, loss of items or loss of direction

Stage 4 – (Moderate cognitive decline) memory deficits in task completion and events –
Time and person orientation may still be present, but the ability to travel alone or function alone may be difficult. Denial of condition is strong.

Stage 5 – (Moderately severe cognitive decline) early dementia when patients need assistance to manage daily functions –
Disorientation to time, place, and people is present, but information about personal facts may be intact. Clothing choices may be a problem, but toileting and eating are usually done independently.

Stage 6 – (Severe cognitive decline) the middle stage of dementia evidenced by lack of ability to remember key people or recent events –
Dependence on caregivers is acute, and most daily activities require assistance. Emotional upheavals and personality changes are present.

Stage 7 – (Very severe cognitive decline) loss of verbal and speech abilities –
Incontinence is present, and there is a need for feeding. Brain connections needed for skills such as walking may no longer be present.

Is Alzheimer's contagious? It's possible. It is not proven that you can catch it from someone already affected by the disease, but some of the latest studies suggest Alzheimer's MIGHT (not proven conclusively) be related to an infection acquired through the nose – possibly a virus or bacteria that is inhaled and travels to the olfactory bulb and into the hippocampus. The brain mounts an immune response to the infection using its own technique that results in the formation of free radicals and plaques, which then cause a cascade of problems as the free radicals damage nearby neurons and create increasing numbers of plaques. This theory comes from an unpublished report by Rudolf Tanzi at Harvard, and he may be onto something. Tanzi doesn't yet know which specific infection initiates Alzheimer's, but studies in mouse brains have shown Alzheimer's-like effects when their brains are infected with viruses. Tanzi's new theory, announced in April 2012 when visiting the University of Southern California (USC), revolutionizes our thinking about Alzheimer's.

Alzheimer's is easily confused with other dementias. From a service perspective, the differences tend to be less important than from a clinician's standpoint, where the treatments and prognosis are highly dependent on the reason for the dementia. Focusing on dementia for now, we know that having high blood pressure is a risk factor for dementia. High blood pressure is often found in those with senile plaques, neurofibrillary tangles, and hippocampal atrophy, though it's certainly not a causal mechanism. Hypertension is also a risk factor for stroke, ischemic white matter lesions, silent infarcts, and general atherosclerosis, which can all lead to dementia as well. In addition, high blood pressure often clusters with other vascular risk factors including diabetes mellitus, obesity, and hypercholesterolemia. These risk factors have also been related to Alzheimer's disease.

Regarding Alzheimer's specifically, several studies have reported that blood pressure is increased in persons with Alzheimer's disease (AD) decades before the recognized onset of the disease. Just a few years before diagnosis, retrospective analyses have shown that blood pressure often declines and continues to decrease during the disease process. Several observational studies have reported that the use of antihypertensive drugs might decrease the risk of Alzheimer's disease.

Regarding the genetics of the disease, substantial efforts have been invested to identify the genetic risk factors underlying Alzheimer's. The only firmly established risk factor remains the ε4 (E4) allele of the apolipoprotein E gene (APOE). If a person has that gene, which is quite rare, they have a 50% higher chance of developing Alzheimer's than if they had one of the other three types of that gene. Many people are developing dense maps of single-nucleotide polymorphisms (SNPs) and large-scale genetic studies, but so far APOE E4 is the big one. That gene is related to brain immune function – supporting Tanzi's idea that perhaps it is an infection that leads to Alzheimer's disease. In addition, mice with the E4 gene have stronger immune responses in the brain. Although a stronger immune response may appear to be a good thing, the immune system the brain uses causes a lot of collateral damage. The immune system takes the 'nuclear approach' with a huge response that damages a greater area when attacking what could be a small infection.

For a little more on the symptoms people show before and after diagnosis, the graph on the following page illustrates that behavioral symptoms appear at all stages of Alzheimer's disease – sometimes as early as three years prior to diagnosis. While individual symptoms can vary tremendously, the overall prevalence of disturbances observed in one study are indicated on a timeline of disease progression.

Social withdrawal was observed in this study an average of 33 months before diagnosis, and was the earliest recognizable psychiatric symptom observed in this study. Suicidal ideation, depression, paranoia, and diurnal rhythm disturbances also occurred early in the course of the disease, whereas agitation, hallucinations, and aggression tend to be found an average of one to two years after diagnosis.

Behavioral Symptoms as AD Progresses

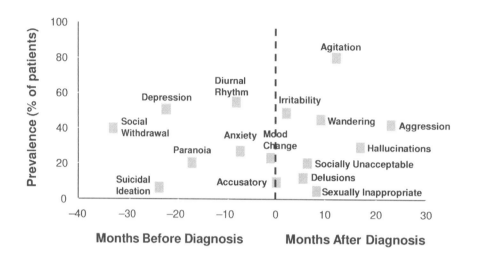

Jost BC, Grossberg GT. *J Am Geriatr Soc.* 1996;44:1078-1081.

Additional Information Concerning Types of Dementias

Dementia with Lewy Bodies (DLB) is another of the most common types of dementia. The symptoms can include staring into space, disorganized speech, drowsiness, and lethargy. This disease is caused by a buildup of Lewy Bodies. Individuals with this disease might have visual hallucinations, depression or a loss of spontaneous movement. These buildups are found in the part of the brain that controls different aspects of memory and motor control. Sometimes medication can assist with the motor symptoms and the psychotic symptoms.

Vascular Dementia can be determined by an autopsy. Multi-Infract Dementia (MID) is a type of vascular dementia caused by multiple strokes that affect the brain. Blood clots in the brain lead to death of brain tissue. Diabetes and high blood pressure, which can cause MID, are both treatable. Many of the symptoms of MID include poor cognitive and motor function, inappropriate social behavior, depression, migraines, incontinence, hallucinations, and memory loss.

Frontotemporo Dementia (FTD), also known as Pick's disease, is the shrinkage of certain parts of the brain due to loss or damage of nerve cells and their connectors. This disease shows similar symptoms to Alzheimer's, dementia with Lewy Bodies, and Huntington's disease. This disease involves a disturbance with an individual's behavior and personality, and causes a person to be restless and antisocial in their actions. As this disease progresses, the individual may have trouble swallowing and experience an increased difficulty in breathing. This disease can develop in younger individuals and last for a number of years.

Binswanger's Dementia is a neurological disease that affects the frontal lobes of the brain. This dementia involves hypertension and intellectual impairment, mood swings, personality changes, and mood swings that become increasingly worse as the disease progresses.

Parkinson's Disease typically starts between the age of 50 and 60. It is a degenerative disease that becomes progressively worse. The first symptoms include the shaking of the hands and/or head. These movements can stop when a person is engaged in meaningful activity or is distracted. As the disease progresses, the person may have difficulty changing positions and talking. Facial expressions take on a flat affect and their posture changes to be more forward. Initially the person experiences forgetfulness, then they may have increased episodes of confusion, paranoia, and irritability. Several physical issues also occur including drier skin around facial features, problems swallowing, and difficulty with urination.

Introduction to Personality Disorders

Personality Disorders: Schizotypal, Antisocial and Schizophrenia

Schizotypal personality disorder is grouped into Cluster A personality disorders, along with other disorders that are similar such as paranoid and schizoid. People with Cluster A disorders exhibit odd or eccentric behavior including distrust of others and a detachment from others (Butcher, pg. 376). People with this disorder behave as introverts. In addition to being socially inhibited, they also have cognitive and perceptual distortions when they communicate with others. Individuals with this disorder seem to maintain an orderly life; however they tend to exhibit a suspicious nature – even to the extreme of believing that they possess magical powers (Butcher, pg. 380). Individuals may think that simple gestures mean something significant when they really don't. Often the person's speech is odd or takes on an odd tone – not to the point of being extremely obvious or disruptive, but in a paranoid kind of manner. Thought patterns are altered, which affect their speech and behaviors. The *Diagnostic and Statistical Manual of Mental Disorders* (*DSM*) criteria includes odd beliefs, inappropriate constricted affect, lack of close friends, and excessive social anxiety (Butcher, pg. 379).

An antisocial personality disorder (ASPD) occurs in the B Cluster, which includes other disorders such as Histrionic, Narcissistic, and Borderline personalities. People with antisocial disorders are said to have a lack of moral or ethical development; they can be very deceitful, and behave in a manner which is socially unacceptable. Those individuals who are antisocial have had issues stemming from early childhood. This disorder affects males more than females at a ratio of 3 to 1. People suffering with this disorder often violate the rights of others. They show deceit and disrespect toward others through aggressive, antisocial behavior. They can also be impulsive and irritable (Butcher, pg. 385).

"Schizophrenia is a severe psychiatric disorder with a broad impact on all aspects of personal, social, and vocational functioning" (Hersen, M. & Thomas, J. C., 2002). People who suffer from this disorder have great difficulty keeping a job, let alone maintaining anything long term. Signs and symptoms of schizophrenia generally are divided into three categories – positive, negative, and cognitive.

In schizophrenia, positive symptoms reflect an excess or distortion of normal functions. The positive symptoms of this disorder are hallucinations, delusions, and other bizarre behaviors. Negative symptoms refer to a diminishment or absence of characteristics of normal function. They may appear with or without positive symptoms. Negative symptoms include "anhedonia (diminished experience of pleasure), asociality (reduced social drive), anergia (decreased ability to initiate and follow through with plans), alogia (poverty of speech or content of speech), and blunted affect (diminished emotional expressiveness)." Cognitive symptoms involve problems with thought processes. These symptoms may be the most disabling in schizophrenia because they interfere with the ability to perform routine daily tasks. A person with schizophrenia may be born with these symptoms, which include problems with making sense of information, difficulty paying attention and memory problems (Hersen, M. & Thomas, J. C., 2002).

Theories of Biological Aging

By definition, a theory integrates known information and explains why events occur in the natural world. Any given theory should be testable and should predict future behaviors. A theory is usually stated as a relationship between two concepts such as age and involvement in the social world. One concept is an independent event (e.g., age), and the other is a dependent event (e.g., social involvement), for which we can explain the reason for its occurrence.

In gerontology, theorists try their best to explain the social behaviors of older adults based on observational evidence. They then develop an explanation and test whether their explanation can predict a prior behavior.

Many theories exist regarding why we age. Some of the more common theories include wear and tear theory, theories involving immune function, cross-linkage theory, free radical theory, and the cellular aging theory.

The wear and tear theory states that aging is a programmed process with a biological clock and a maximum life span. Theorists have studied and observed animal species as evidence for this theory. Many insects live for just a few days, no matter how perfect their environment. The cells of living bodies simply wear out over time, and damaged cells cannot be repaired fast enough.

Some body cells such as heart and nerve cells are not usually replaced in adults – even after severe damage – and this damage accumulates. Although this theory is a little simplistic, it offers some ideas that appear to be plausible.

Autoimmune theory proposes that aging is a function of the decline in the immune system. With age, the body becomes more susceptible to infection. This increases the risk of cancer, diabetes, and rheumatoid arthritis. The thymus gland, where white blood cells are made, shrinks with age. This theory does not explain why the immune system deteriorates, and it doesn't apply to all older people since autoimmune diseases are not universal.

Cross-linkage theory focuses on the protein collagen, an important connective tissue found in most organs. Collagen is very abundant in our body and accounts for about one third of the protein in our body. As we age, collagen production declines. This leads to more wrinkles, a decline in the elasticity of blood vessels, a decrease in muscle tissue, and even a decline in the flexibility of the eye lens, leading to increased farsightedness with aging. Changes in the collagen proteins associated with aging are caused by increased binding of molecules in the cells of older organisms, which slows normal cell functions.

The free radical theory states that the normal use of oxygen in metabolism results in a creation of highly reactive molecules with an unpaired electron. The unpaired electron causes molecules to seek out an electron from neighboring atoms (usually taking away an electron from a nearby molecule), which results in a chain reaction of electron exchange. The damage caused to the body by this process is referred to as oxidative damage. Over time, oxidative damage accumulates in our bodies and may cause many of the changes associated with biological aging. The body has chemical inhibitors to absorb extra electrons and antioxidants such as vitamin E, vitamin C, beta-carotene, and selenium to further reduce these types of chemical reactions. Normal chemical reactions create these free radicals at low levels, however higher levels are found in people who smoke or are exposed to radiation or psychological stress. The free radicals interact with molecules and can cause DNA mutations, increased cross-linking of connective tissue, and can interfere with protein functions.

Cellular senescence refers to the process through which a cell becomes incapable of dividing due to the influence of an external stimulus, and has been linked to the aging process. Among other factors, the senescence response has been associated with the behavior of cells, specifically with the process of apoptosis. Apoptosis is the deliberate, programmed death of cells. In this process, unwanted extra or damaged cells are removed in a controlled fashion. This prevents the cells from damaging both neighboring cells and the organism itself. It has been hypothesized that a defect in the control of apoptosis is associated with senescence, or the degenerative processes in the body that occur as organisms age. It is currently unclear how this occurs, but it has been suggested that:

1. The apoptotic response decreases as people age, altering an organism's ability to remove unwanted cells, or

2. As organisms age, their ability to compensate for cell loss due to apoptosis (particularly the loss of neurons) is compromised.

One way in which cells know how old they are is through telomeres. Telomeres are extra coding indicators that appear at the beginning and end of each DNA strand and do not code for important proteins. These extra nucleotides are longer in younger people and shorter in older people. This code works like the ends of a shoelace. You can do without the very end of the shoelace, but as the shoelace gets shorter and shorter, eventually it gets too short to be considered useful. Each time the DNA is copied, the DNA strand gets a little bit shorter. As the DNA gradually shortens, important information is eventually lost, leading to an improperly functioning cell. Much research in this area focuses on telomerase, an enzyme associated with the lengthening and repair of telomeres.

Immunosenescence focuses on the decline in the immune system that occurs with aging and increases the risk and susceptibility of infectious disease and death. Some centenarians have highly effective immune responses. However, infectious causes are the primary cause of death in people over 80. At this age, there is a decline in the production of T-cells, B-cells, and lymphocytes. These cells normally create antibodies and serve as the primary and secondary response of immune system needs. Altered immune function in old age may be linked to prostate and skin cancers as well as cardiovascular disease.

Theories of Psychological Aging

Two of the most common psychological theories of aging include that of Maslow's Hierarchy of Needs and Erickson's Eight Stages of Life. However, several other theories include The Continuity Theory, The Activity Theory, and The Disengagement Theory.

Maslow's Hierarchy of Needs is a theory in psychology proposed by Abraham Maslow in a 1943 paper *A Theory of Human Motivation*. His theory on aging parallels many other theories of human developmental psychology, some of which focus on describing the stages of growth in humans. Maslow used the terms Physiological, Safety, Love and Belongingness, Esteem, Self-actualization, also referred to as Self-Transcendence to describe the patterns through which human motivations generally move.

Physiological – Physiological needs are the physical requirements for human survival. If these requirements are not met, the human body cannot function properly and will ultimately fail. Physiological needs are thought to be the most important, and should be met first. These physiological needs include air, water, food, clothing, and shelter.

Safety – Once physical needs are met, a person then focuses on their feelings of safety from war, disaster, abuse, violence, and conflict. This may include personal, financial, and a healthy sense of security.

Love and Belongingness – The third level of human needs involves feelings of belongingness. This need is especially strong in childhood and involves the individual's ability to form and maintain emotionally significant relationships in general including friendship, intimacy, families, and social groups.

Esteem – Esteem emerges when love and belongingness needs are met. All humans have a need to feel respected. Esteem is one's desire to be accepted and valued by others. Generally people engage in a profession or hobby to gain recognition. These activities give the person a sense of contribution or value. Low self-esteem or an inferiority complex may result from imbalances during this level in the hierarchy.

Self-actualization – A self-actualized person has a realistic perception of both themselves and others. They know their strengths, weaknesses, and limitations, and are able to see others and events realistically. This person doesn't just accept things on face value; they are able to problem solve, and set and accomplish goals. Independence, self-motivation, and spontaneity are some of the traits of a self-actualized individual.

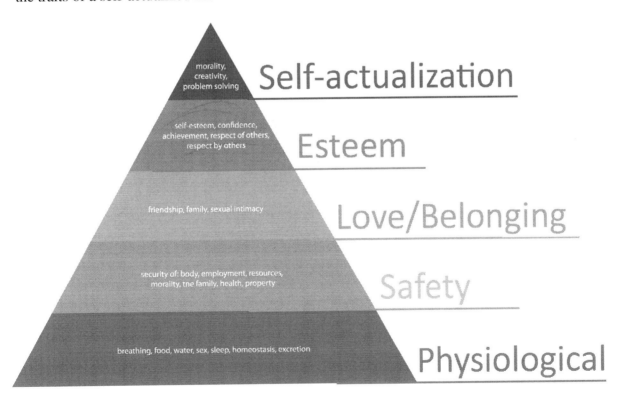

Maslow's Hierarchy of Needs

Erickson's Eight Stages of Life

Erik Erickson developed a theory that involves eight stages experienced in human life. His theory stated that a person develops their personality by the way they resolve various life stages. Results can be either positive or negative, and there can be a varying degree of resolution in life situations – depending on how individuals resolve issues encountered throughout life.

Stage 1: Infancy – Age 0 to 1

Crisis: Trust vs. Mistrust

Description: In the first year of life, infants depend on others for food, warmth, and affection, and therefore must be able to blindly trust parents (or caregivers) for providing those basic needs.

Positive outcome: If needs are met consistently and responsively by the parents, infants will not only develop a secure attachment with parents, but will also learn to trust their environment in general.

Negative outcome: If needs are not met consistently and responsively, infants will develop mistrust toward people and their environment – even toward themselves.

Stage 2: Toddler – Age 1 to 2

Crisis: Autonomy (Independence) vs. Doubt (or Shame)

Description: Toddlers learn to walk, talk, use toilets, and do things for themselves. Their self-control and self-confidence begin to develop at this stage.

Positive outcome: If parents encourage their child's use of initiative and reassure her when she makes mistakes, the child will develop the confidence needed to cope with future situations that require choice, control, and independence.

Negative outcome: If parents are overprotective, or disapproving of the child's acts of independence, he may begin to feel ashamed of his behavior or doubt his own abilities.

Stage 3: Early Childhood – Age 2 to 6

Crisis: Initiative vs. Guilt

Description: Children have newfound power at this stage as they have developed motor skills and have become increasingly engaged in social interaction with people around them. They now must learn to achieve a balance between eagerness for more adventure and responsibility and learning to control impulses and childish fantasies.

Positive outcome: If parents are encouraging, but consistent in discipline, children will learn to accept without guilt that certain behaviors are not allowed. At the same time, they shouldn't feel shame when using imagination and engaging in make-believe role-playing.

Negative outcome: If parents are not encouraging, and are inconsistent with discipline, children may develop a sense of guilt and may come to believe that it is wrong to be independent.

Stage 4: Elementary and Middle School Years – Age 6 to 12

Crisis: Competence (Industry) vs. Inferiority

Description: School is the important event at this stage. Children learn to make things, use tools, and acquire the skills to be a worker and a potential provider all while making the transition from the world of home into the world of peers.

Positive outcome: If children can discover pleasure in intellectual stimulation, being productive, and seeking success, they will develop a sense of competence.

Negative outcome: If children do not achieve intellectual stimulation or find success, they will develop a sense of inferiority.

Stage 5: Adolescence – Age 12 to 18

Crisis: Identity vs. Role Confusion

Description: This is the time when children ask the question, "Who am I?" To successfully answer this question, Erikson suggests adolescents must integrate the healthy resolution of all earlier conflicts: developing a basic sense of trust, building a strong sense of independence, gaining competence, and feeling in control of their life. Adolescents who have successfully dealt with earlier conflicts are ready for the 'Identity Crisis,' which is considered by Erikson as the most significant conflict a person must face.

Positive outcome: If the adolescent solves this conflict successfully, they will exit this stage with a strong identity and readiness to plan for the future.

Negative outcome: If adolescents do not solve conflicts successfully, they will sink into confusion, unable to make decisions and choices, especially about vocation, sexual orientation, and life roles.

Stage 6: Young Adulthood – Age 19 to 40

Crisis: Intimacy vs. Isolation

Description: In this stage, the most important events are love relationships. No matter how successful you are with your work, said Erikson, you are not developmentally complete until you are capable of intimacy. An individual who has not developed a sense of identity usually will fear a committed relationship and may retreat into isolation.

Positive outcome: Adult individuals can form close relationships and share with others if they have achieved a sense of identity.

Negative outcome: If adults do not form close relationships, they will fear commitment, feel isolated, and be unable to depend on anybody in the world.

Stage 7: Middle Adulthood – Age 40 to 65

Crisis: Generativity vs. Stagnation

Description: By *generativity*, Erikson refers to the adult's ability to look outside oneself and care for others (e.g., through parenting). Erikson suggests that adults need children as much as children need adults, and that this stage reflects the need to create a living legacy.

Positive outcome: People can solve this crisis by having and nurturing children or helping the next generation in other ways.

Negative outcome: If adults are unable to develop empathy and compassion by caring for and understanding others, the person will remain self-centered and experience stagnation later in life.

Stage 8: Late Adulthood – Age 65 to death

Crisis: Integrity vs. Despair Important

Description: Old age is a time for reflecting upon one's own life and its role in the big scheme of things, and either seeing it filled with pleasure and satisfaction or disappointment and failure.

Positive outcome: If adults have achieved a sense of fulfillment about life and a sense of unity within themselves and with others, they will accept death with a sense of integrity. Just as the healthy child will not fear life, said Erikson, the healthy adult will not fear death.

Negative outcome: If adults do not achieve that sense of fulfillment about life, they will despair and fear death.

The Continuity Theory was developed by Robert Atchley in 1972. It is based on ideas from Bernice Neugarten, Vern L. Bengtson's teacher at the University of Chicago, in 1968. (Bengtson has published 16 books and 260 research papers on gerontology, theories of aging, sociology of aging and family sociology. All theorists used in today's teachings knew each other well and cooperated to some extent in the development of their ideas.) The continuity theory emphasizes that personality plays a major role in adjustment to aging and that adult development is a continuous process. According to continuity theory, individuals tend to maintain a stable and consistent pattern of behavior as they get older. When older people are forced to relinquish one role (e.g., employee), they try to substitute similar roles for the lost role (e.g., volunteering or starting a hobby). People try not to create or experience change dramatically and, in fact, base their life satisfaction on how consistent they can be from year to year.

Robert Havinghurst formalized the Activity Theory in 1969. According to this theory, life satisfaction is highest among older people who are active and busy. Our concept of who we are as a person (in sociology, termed sense of self or self-concept) is validated through participation in the same or similar substitute roles and activities that middle-aged people participate in. According to this theory, older people who lose one role (e.g., losing a spouse) usually replace it with another role (e.g., adopting a dog or joining a social group).

Elaine Cumming and William Henry, two researchers at the University of Chicago, proposed the disengagement theory in 1961. They noted that 'normal aging,' from their perspective, involves a natural and inevitable mutual withdrawal or disengagement that results in decreasing social interaction between the aging person and society. The authors reasoned that the elderly gradually lose interest in life as they prepare for death. The evidence for this is manifested in shrinking social contacts and less interest in social participation. Cumming and Henry proposed that this process is universal, inevitable, and intrinsic. In other words, it is a natural process that happens to all older adults regardless of culture. They proposed that this process is necessary and beneficial for society because this process lessens disruptions (within the family, the workplace, and other societal structures) upon the death of an older adult.

Arnold Rose applied Subculture Theory to the study of aging. According to this theory, subcultures develop when people share similar interests, problems, and concerns or have long-standing friendships and are excluded from full participation in wider society. We see this phenomenon often today in social groups using the Internet to band people together who share common interests, in religious groups hosting very active social schedules, or in ethnic-centered social groups.

This theory states that an aging subculture developed for two reasons:

1. Older adults shared common interests and experiences (e.g., failing health, generational experience, common life stage).

2. Older adults are excluded from full participation in wider society (e.g., older adults encouraged to socialize in age-segregated institutions such as senior centers or move to age-segregated housing such as retirement communities).

The Exchange theory grew from micro-economics theory. This theory posits that interaction between the old and young decrease because older people have fewer resources to bring to the exchange – lower income or income potential, poorer health, and less relevant education. However, this theory ignores the value of nonrational resources (e.g., love and companionship) and focuses on immediate interaction between older people and other age groups.

Modernization Theory (Cowgill & Holmes, 1972) evolved from the optimism which characterized the United States in the post-World War II era. The theory asserts that the elderly status is inversely related to the level of societal modernization. With increasing modernization (advanced health technology, economic development, increasing education, urbanization), the status of elderly individuals inevitably declines. Cowgill later revised this theory to postulate that there may be a bottoming out of elderly status and perhaps an improvement in their social status as society ages.

Age stratification theory is one of the most influential and enduring gerontological theories. Matilda W. Riley (1971) proposed this theory, which focuses on structural, demographic, and historical influences in late-life satisfaction. On the micro level, this theory argues that age is the basis for sense of self in the social world. At the macro level, we can study how changes in the age structure of society over time affects our expectations on older people. The theory notes that all societies group people into social categories based on age, and these groupings provide major social identities. Life satisfaction (the dependent factor) is a function of the interactions and expectations with others, and these interactions and expectations are highly influenced by age. When studying elderly life satisfaction, we must account for age and birth cohort because of their influence on the way an individual thinks, behaves, and expects to contribute to society.

Political Economy Theories see the elderly as helpless to the environment in which they live. Social class (i.e., limited resources) forms a barrier to social resources like political power because those with political power perpetuate social inequality to maintain authority. So it is the socioeconomic and political environment that shape your old age experience, which is constrained by social class, gender, and ethnicity.

Physiological Aging

Everyone is slightly different in their physiological changes, but these are common trends. The water content of cells declines with age. For men, the proportion of body weight that is water drops from 60% to 54%; for women, this proportion drops from 52% to 46%. Body tissues and muscles become thinner with age, leading to relative increases in the portion of fat in the body. The age-associated weakening of muscles is sometimes called sarcopenia. After age 50, the number of muscle fibers declines. By age 80, just over half of the muscle fibers from the mid-twenties remain. Exercise can slow down this process.

Drugs are an important aspect of senior health care. The increase in fat, decrease in muscle, and decrease in water are some reasons that medications sometimes work differently in the elderly. Medications vary, but some are processed by muscle tissue, some in water, and some in fat. Doctors need to take this into account when considering dosage for older patients.

Adults also experience a reduction in height beginning at age 30 – about 1/16 inches per year in both the trunk and extremities through the loss of bone mineral. The spine becomes more curved and the vertebrae discs become more compacted. In cases of osteoporosis, bone loss is more severe, therefore increasing the risk of fractures – even during a minor stress.

Kyphosis is the additional hunch in the neck that occurs in older people due to crush fractures. The cartilage between the joints gets thinner with availability of less lubricating fluid.

Touch sensitivity declines with aging. There are changes in the skin and nerve endings, leading to lower distinction between levels of pain and potentially more serious burns due to delayed response.

Maximum breathing capacity requires coordination of the respiratory, nervous, and muscular systems, and is greatly impacted by the aging process. The muscles controlling the lungs lose both elasticity and efficiency. Vital capacity, the maximum amount of oxygen that can be inhaled with a deep breath, declines by 50% between the mid-twenties and early seventies. This can lead to decreased ability to exercise and further muscle decline. With exercise, the muscles that control breathing can be maintained, thereby reducing the decline in breathing capacity, though not totally eliminating the effects of aging.

Cilia, hairlike projections in the airway, normally filter foreign matter from the air, but their functionality also gradually declines with age. This decline in function increases the risk of respiratory conditions such as chronic bronchitis, emphysema, and pneumonia.

Structural changes in the heart occur in older age when muscle is replaced with fat, elastic tissue declines, and collagen increases. The arteries become stiffer, and swelling due to high pressure can occur in the veins, leading to varicose veins. Atherosclerosis refers to the artery walls becoming increasingly lined with lipids, decreasing the amount of blood that can travel through the vessels.

When under strain, the older heart pumps harder rather than faster. This change in heart function can lead to greater efficiency; however it can also lead to higher blood pressure. With age, the risk for systolic blood pressure increases as does the resting heart rate, however both conditions can be controlled to some extent through exercise.

The kidneys are the organs most affected by aging. Kidneys decrease in both volume and weight, resulting in a decline of about 50% in filtering function. This decline can have a great impact on tolerance, and extends the active period for medications such as penicillin, tetracycline, and other drugs. Kidneys also lose the ability to absorb glucose, contributing to problems of dehydration and a loss of salt in the blood. The bladder can also lose 50% of its capacity with extreme old age, and the sensation of needing to use the restroom is delayed, increasing the risk of urinary incontinence. Caffeine and alcohol can exasperate the effects of these disorders.

Social Demographics of Aging

Demography is the science of population – the mathematical study of a population's characteristics. Formal demography focuses on the size, distribution, structure, and change of populations. Size and distribution refer to the arrangement of the population in a given space and time (geographically or by type of residential area). Structure refers to categories of description such as sex, race, and age (also marital and family status, place of birth, literacy, education level, or similar category). Change refers to growth or decline of any given category (also referred to as structural unit) over a defined time period.

Population aging refers to an increase in the proportion of older adults within an overall population. The past century has been marked by rapid population aging both within the U.S. and globally. This growth has often been associated with doomsday scenarios in which frail older adults will overwhelm our society.

In conjunction with the R.O.S. Therapy Systems program, the focus will mostly cover the growth of the 65 and older population. A baby boom exists in almost every population pyramid, but the relative change in the ratio of young to old leads to population aging.

The charts on the next page indicate roughly the number of people who will be eligible to participate in certain government programs such as Medicare and Social Security. This number has already increased dramatically over the last 100 years, and will continue to increase rapidly in the first part of this century.

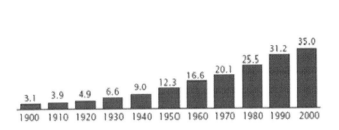

Figure 2-1.
Population Aged 65 and Over: 1900 to 2000
(In millions)

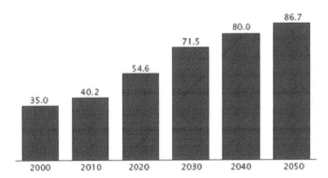

Figure 2-5.
Population Aged 65 and Over: 2000 to 2050
(In millions)

Figure taken from 65+ in the United States, 2005; U.S. Census Bureau Publication #P23-209

The percentage of the population that is older than 65 has also been growing for about 100 years. As shown in the charts below, the percent of the U.S. population over the age of 65 has increased from 4.1% in 1900 to 12.4% in 2000. By 2050, adults over age 65 are projected to make up more than one-fifth of our population.

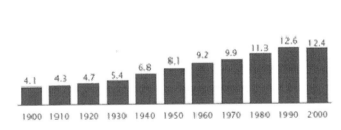

Figure 2-2.
Percent Aged 65 and Over of the Total Population: 1900 to 2000

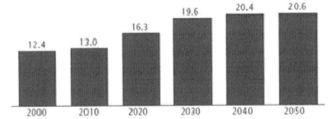

Figure 2-6.
Percent Aged 65 and Over of the Total Population: 2000 to 2050

Figure taken from 65+ in the United States: 2005; U.S. Census Bureau Publication # P23-209

Life Expectancy and Life Span

This change in the proportion of older adults is due primarily to changes in life expectancy over the same period. Life expectancy is defined as the average number of years an individual within a particular geographic region, country, gender, or race/ethnicity is expected to live. In other words, if the average life expectancy of a particular population is 80 years, half of those in the population will die before age 80, while the other half will die after age 80.

Usually life expectancy is calculated at birth; however life expectancy can be calculated from any age. Most commonly, life expectancy is calculated from age 65. Life expectancy at 65 is the estimated number of years you can expect to live if you have already lived to age 65. While the average life expectancy at birth in 1900 was only 47.3 years, for those who reached age 65 life expectancy became nearly 77 years. In 2000, those who reached age 65 could expect, on average, to live to age 83.

Life span, different from life expectancy, is the maximum age a member of a species can attain. The life span of humans is projected to be approximately 120 years. The longest proven human life span is attributed to Jeanne Louise Calment, a French woman from the village of Arles. She was born on February 21, 1875, and died in August 1997, at the age of 122 years, 164 days. However, controversy does exist regarding Calment's record. Some reports say that numerous other individuals may have lived longer, yet records were not maintained to verify these facts, especially in third world countries.

Why Does the Age Structure of a Population Matter?

If people did exactly the same thing at all ages or had exactly the same needs and abilities at all ages, the age structure of the population would not make much difference. The relevance of the age structure is based on the fact that people of different ages have different needs, abilities, responsibilities, and entitlements. Some population structure changes relate to biological changes that correlate with chronological age. For instance, it would not be possible for very young children to survive without the help of older members of society. Children need to be taught to become self-sufficient. It is also possible that a small number of very elderly and infirm people could not survive without the help of younger members of society.

On the whole, however, the importance of age differences arise because of societal expectations and societal circumstances that determine what one does and what one is entitled to at a given age. Very few people younger than age 20 support themselves because many remain in school after that age – not because of a physical need to be dependent, but because an advanced technological society requires extensive training before undertaking many career positions. At the other end of the age range, most people over the age of 64 receive some government support in the form of Social Security income and medical care under the government sponsored program of Medicare. These programs exist not because of some physical necessity linked to age, but because of societal arrangements whereby entitlement to certain programs is linked to age. The meaning of the age composition of a country is thus determined in part by social and political arrangements in that country.

Compression of Morbidity

Are older adults surviving previous 'killer' diseases, such as heart attack and stroke, at a greater rate only to live with chronic illness and disability? This interesting and important question has been raised as life expectancy has increased. Part of this issue relates to the concepts of the compression of mortality and its effects on morbidity.

In 1980, Dr. James Fries wrote a compelling article that hypothesized the possibility to lower rates of morbidity (the burden of disease) while extending life expectancy. The article proposed multiple scenarios. The first scenario, or the extension of morbidity, would occur if life expectancy increased, but the age of disease onset stayed stable (or increased at a slower rate than life expectancy). This shift would increase the total number of years spent with high levels of morbidity. Second, a shift to the right could occur in which life expectancy and the age of disease onset increase at the same rate. In this case, people would live longer and experience the first onset of disease later, but the total number of years spent with disease and disability would still remain the same. Finally, a compression of morbidity could occur in which the age of illness onset increased at a faster rate than life expectancy. In this case, older adults would live longer and with fewer years of disease and disability.

BRIEF Introduction to Home Care

Home care may be utilized for persons living alone or arranged by a person or family member. Professional, licensed caregivers advertise services according to their license. Non-professional or non-licensed caregivers generally advertise services as personal care such as providing companionship, performing light housekeeping or offering transportation to doctor appointments, and other such services.

As home health care is increasingly becoming a sought-after service, older adults will be able to remain in their homes longer with assistance in daily activities (ADLs). All caregivers provide various degrees of socialization to the client. A variety of programs have been developed to assist with providing quality life experiences among the activities of daily living, which will be addressed later in this how-to manual.

As the need for home health care increases, so will the need for in-home activities. Many activities are available and can be divided into three categories: independent activities (can perform on one's own with supplies), group activities (can perform with two or more other individuals such as neighbors, roommates or friends), and individualized activities (can be developed and implemented on a one-on-one basis).

<u>Independent activities</u> include watching television, listening to music, reading the newspaper, praying, reading, writing letters, solving puzzles and word games, and creating simple crafts.

<u>Group activities</u> can include playing board games, cards, and other activities requiring two or more individuals.

<u>Individualized activities</u> are generally conducted between a family member and a loved one when the loved one is not receiving any type of personal care (grooming, meals or ADLs) or between the home health aide and client. Individualized activities are one-on-one activities that might center on the family, life review, current events or something specific to the person's interests. For example, if the loved one enjoyed horses, a family member/caregiver could look at photos of horses with their loved one/client.

Providing the proper supplies and equipment, supporting the client/loved one through listening and prayer, and participating in other activities along with acquiring proper tools and training can play a key factor in providing quality life experiences for everyone.

Resources

1. The Handbook of Theories on Aging (Bengtson et al., 2009).

2. Activity Keeps Me Going, Volume A (Peckham et al., 2011).

3. Essentials for the Activity Professional in Long-Term Care (Lanza, 1997).

4. Abnormal Psychology (Butcher).

5. "Behavior…Whose Problem Is It?" Hommel, 2012

Section II

Communicating and Motivating for Success

Effective Communication Methods

The key to effective communication in every situation is the ability to listen attentively. This requires the health professional to use communication techniques that provide an open, non-threatening environment for the client. The client must feel free to discuss their problems, issues or concerns. Communicating with the client in a facilitative, nonauthoritative manner (made easier by asking appropriate questions) allows for the smooth, effective exchange of information. Research has shown that using facilitative communication techniques does not take additional time or result in less information than more conventional, direct methods of questioning.

<u>Guidelines to Effective Communication</u>

Use open-ended questions.

Questions that begin with who, what, where, how much, and how often or statements such as, "Tell me more about..." are examples of open-ended questions. These types of questions often elicit more spontaneous information from the client rather than the answer that the client thinks the individual is looking for.

Avoid directed or leading questions.

Direct questions – those with a "Yes" or "No" response – or those which lead a client to give a particular answer should be avoided. The client begins to wonder, "Why ask that?" or "What would he or she want me to answer?"

Use clarification questions when the client provides vague information.

The client may use words like "sometimes" or "occasionally" to qualify an answer, or they may use words like "bothersome" or "upset" to describe a feeling. The meanings that these words have for the client may be different from the meaning that the listener is attaching to them. A failure to ask for clarification could create problems when trying to completely understand the situation. It is also often difficult for the client to describe a feeling or a sensation. It is equally important that the listener help the client in this case.

Show warmth and understanding by nonverbal actions and statements that reflect the client's feelings.

Warmth is conveyed to another person by eye contact, open body posture, appropriate facial expressions, and other nonverbal signs showing interest and attention. Silence is another powerful nonverbal technique, if used correctly. When you really *listen* to the client, you will be less likely to interrupt the person. Also, you may sense when it is better to remain silent rather than immediately ask another question if the client appears hesitant.

Understanding is demonstrated by attending to the client's feelings and concerns. When you acknowledge the client's feelings by paraphrasing what you are hearing, the client realizes that the other person considers this important and that no judgment is being pronounced on these feelings. This type of interaction however runs counter to our traditional practices dealing with the facts.

A few common, but at the same time harmful, ways of responding to such expressions of the client are to offer a false reassurance or use jargon. Saying "Don't worry about that" or "It will all work out" are examples of false reassurances. These statements help the listener avoid dealing with a difficult situation, but are of little help to the client. In fact, it may compound the problem. Quite often, such statements convey a sense of judgment to the client that inhibits future discussions of these feelings or other aspects of the problem related to them. Initially, responding to feelings can feel funny or mechanical, because we're not used to doing it. Like any other skill to be learned, it becomes more comfortable and natural with practice.

The Role of the Listener

The role of the listener is very important, because listening behavior can either enhance and encourage communication or shut down communication altogether. Volunteers need to assess their listening style as well as be able to assess the listening styles of the clients and families with whom they are working.

The types of listeners that run the gamut are: pseudo-listeners, selective listeners, stage huggers, insulated listeners, defensive listeners and ambushers, and insensitive listeners. *Pseudo-listeners'* behavior and body language lead one to believe that they're listening. However, if asked to repeat what was said, most likely the pseudo-listener could not since they were not focused on the speaker. *Selective listeners* hear only what is of interest to them. These listeners tend to *tune out* and only respond to specific remarks. *Stage huggers* are not interested in the speaker or what the speaker has to say. Rather, they're more interested in stating their remarks, thereby dominating the conversation. *Insulated listeners* turn listening off when they do not want to deal with the matter at hand because what is being said often elicits an emotional response. *Defensive listeners* and *ambushers* are usually individuals with low self-esteem who either take what is being said personally and misinterpret the information or use the information against someone at a later time. This type of behavior is passive-aggressive and usually signals someone who is angry. *Insensitive listeners* do not seem to "get it," and they cannot look beyond words or see nonverbal clues.

None of these types of listeners would make an effective volunteer because the one major skill most needed in health care work is the ability to listen well. A lack of communication skills may become apparent when a client or family member is expressing emotional pain. Instead of listening, reflecting, and supporting, a helper unskilled in communication might begin to ask a lot of questions, make inappropriate self-disclosures, dismiss their pain with platitude or give advice. A good listener, on the other hand, is fully present in the moment and emotionally available to the speaker. Listening well involves entering the world of the speaker, encouraging further disclosure, and identifying and validating feelings. It is making a conscious choice to imagine what it is like to be the speaker, communicating in verbal and nonverbal ways that you are open and ready to hear more, and interjecting statements which indicate that you are with them where they are such as, "I can see how that would have been very frustrating" or "You must have been really angry."

Verbal Communication

Communication is an interactive process to exchange information. The ability to respond appropriately and to give feedback on something communicated is just as important as having good listening skills. Sometimes, however, our well-intentioned responses end up hurting rather than helping. Some of the ways that one might respond in an unintentionally hurtful way might be telling clients and family members not to cry or be upset instead of allowing them to express their feelings, drawing on personal experience to give advice, judging or analyzing what was said without clarifying the intended meaning or offering unsolicited tidbits of practical or religious wisdom.

Effective communication involves developing rapport and empathy. It involves being sensitive moment to moment toward someone else's fear, rage, tenderness, confusion or whatever he or she is experiencing. To be a good listener, one must absorb the mood of the other person as well as notice their body language and their affect as nonverbal communication is equally or more important than the words one uses.

Volunteers often feel they need to respond quickly to keep the conversation active so, at times, the end of the sentences is missed and the message is cut short. When responses are formulated slowly, it allows for more time to hear and process the information. When there are times of quiet, it allows both the sender and receiver to experience what is happening at the time. Silence is an appropriate and helpful technique. Silence allows time for people to pull thoughts and ideas together that are often more meaningful.

Process –

1) Establish your willingness to listen.

   Examples of language to utilize
   "I'm listening."
   "I'm here."
   "Would you like to talk about that?"
   "Do you feel like talking about that?"
   "Could you say more about that?"
   "Listening is what I am here for."

2) Recognize the person behind the words, and hear and acknowledge their feelings.

   Examples of language to utilize
   "It sounds like you may be angry."
   "How did it feel when that happened?"
   "You must have felt hurt."
   "Are you still upset when you think about that?"
   "Have you had those feelings other times?"
   "What kind of feelings are you having right now?"

3) Help the person think and discover what they already know or feel and what is going on.

   Examples of language to utilize
   "What ideas have you already considered?"
   "You seem to have several ideas about what would help."
   "How long has this been happening to you?"
   "A minute ago, you said..."
   "Do I hear you saying…?"
   "How do you act when that happens?"

4) Assist the person in beginning the decision-making process.

   Examples of language to utilize
   "How would you like to feel?"
   "What do you feel you should do?"
   "What choices do you have or see?"
   "What do you see as your next step?"
   "What are your plans right now?"

5) Offer information, ideas or insights of your own. Make people aware of referral agencies without trying to solve their problems.

<u>Examples of language to utilize</u>
"Have you ever tried…?"
"Have you heard about...?"
"Did you know…?"
"Have you considered…?"
"I wonder if..."
"Does it seem to you that…?"

6) Help the person put together what happened during your conversation.

<u>Examples of language to utilize</u>
"How do you feel about that now?"
"Are you feeling differently now?"
"Do you understand more about what has happened?"
"What are your plans now?"
"What are you going to do next?"
"Do you know now what you want to work on?"

7) Help the person close the conversation.

<u>Examples of language to utilize</u>
"I hope things will be better for you soon."
"Well, I wish you well with your plans."
"I'm glad that you decided to talk about this."
"Maybe you could talk about this again after you give it more thought."

Communication is an art and how you approach a client will determine whether the interaction produces the outcomes you desire. In Section I, we reviewed the changes experienced throughout aging; because of those multi-system losses, a client's perception of their environment and the people in it hinges on the approaches used in communication.

Successful Communication Approaches

- <u>Be calm</u>: Always approach the client in a relaxed and calm demeanor. Your mood will be mirrored by the client. Smiles are contagious.
- <u>Be flexible</u>: There is no right or wrong way of completing a task. Offer praise and encouragement for the effort a client puts into a task. If you see the client becoming overwhelmed or frustrated, discontinue the task and approach another time.
- <u>Be nonresistive</u>: Don't force tasks on the client. Adults do not want to be told "No" or told what to do. The power of suggestion goes a long way.
- <u>Be guiding, not controlling</u>: Always use a soft, gentle approach, and remember your tone of voice and facial expressions must match your words.

<u>The Wind and the Sun</u>
Æsop (Sixth Century B.C.) Fables.
The Harvard Classics. 1909–14.

The Wind and the Sun were disputing which was the stronger. Suddenly, they saw a traveler coming down the road, and the Sun said: "I see a way to decide our dispute. Whichever of us can cause that traveler to take off his cloak shall be regarded as the stronger. You begin." So the Sun retired behind a cloud, and the Wind began to blow as hard as it could upon the traveler. But the harder he blew, the more closely did the traveler wrap his cloak around him, 'til at last the Wind had to give up in despair. Then the Sun came out and shone in all his glory upon the traveler, who soon found it too hot to walk with his cloak on.

The moral of the story is: "KINDNESS EFFECTS MORE THAN SEVERITY."

This is an example of Successful Communication.

<u>Nonverbal Communication</u>

Although it may seem that most communication happens verbally, research has shown that most communication occurs nonverbally. Nonverbal communication occurs through an individual's body language and facial expressions. Some examples might be:

- Gestures (such as nail biting, hand-wringing, rubbing of head)
- Presence or absence of eye contact (appropriateness of affect)
- Body positioning (arms folded across chest, body facing the other person, or back partially or totally turned away)

Nonverbal communication often sets the stage for the kind of verbal communication that may occur, either for the listener or the sender. The following will help increase volunteers' awareness of the nonverbal messages he or she might be sending.

<u>Attitudes Communicated Nonverbally</u>

Openness

- Hands open
- Coat unbuttoned
- Smile

Defensiveness

- Arms crossed
- Erect posture
- Sitting reversed in an armless chair
- Legs crossed
- Fist-like gestures
- Pointing index fingers
- Karate chops

Evaluation

- Hand-to-face gestures
- Head tilted
- Stroking chin
- Peering over glasses
- Removing glasses … maybe cleaning them
- Getting up from the table and walking around
- Hands on bridge of nose

Suspicion

- Looking away
- Arms crossed
- Moving away
- Sideways glance
- Feet/body leaning or pointing away
- Rubbing eyes or squinting
- Coat buttoned
- Looking or moving toward the exit
- Touching/rubbing nose

Readiness

- Hands on hips
- Hand on mid-thigh when seated
- Sitting on edge of chair
- Arms spread, hands gripping edge of table
- Moving/leaning closer
- Rubbing palms

Self-control

- Hands folded in lap
- Gripping wrists
- Ankles locked
- Hands tightly clenched

Frustration

- Short breaths
- Sighs
- Wringing hands
- Running hands through hair
- Rubbing back of neck
- Eye rolling

Boredom/Impatience

- Doodling
- Finger drumming
- Foot kicking
- Head in palm of hands
- Blank stares
- Foot tapping

Acceptance

- Open arms and hands
- Touching gestures
- Moving/leaning closer
- Head nodding
- Facing an individual
- Smiling

Rejection

- Turning their back
- Giving a 'cold shoulder'
- Tightening jaw muscles

When communicating, 22% of your message comes from words and 78% of your message comes from nonverbal communication. There are five key communication elements to consider: facial expressions, eye contact, gestures and touch, tone of voice, and body language.

Facial Expressions – Be aware of what your facial expressions convey to a client. Remember, your mood will be mirrored. Are you happy, tense, impatient or distracted? When reading a client's facial expressions, what are they trying to tell you? Are they sad, happy or agitated? Look for physical clues beyond their words.

Eye Contact – Always remember to have eye contact, and that the client is focused on you and what you are saying.

Gestures and Touch – Use nonverbal signs such as pointing, waving or universal gestures in combination with words. If you want to ask a client if they are cold, you can say, "Are you cold?" At the same time, place your arms around yourself and rub your upper arms to indicate cold. This technique should be used when listening to a client. Now ask yourself, "What is their gesture saying?"

Tone of Voice – You are paid to have a pleasant tone of voice and a good work attitude. Your reflection in your voice helps your client relate to your words. If your tone indicates that you are rushed or impatient, then your client is less likely to be responsive to the task at hand.

Body Language – Be aware of your hand and arm position when talking to your clients. If your hands are on your hip or if your hands are folded in front of you, you could be perceived as aggressive or judgmental. Consequently, the client will begin to harbor fear or distrust, resulting in an uncooperative client.

Successful communication translates into respect including comfort and care for the client's feelings.

Remember – "People will forget what you said, people will forget what you did, but they will never forget how you made them feel." – Maya Angelou

Communicating with Clients with Challenging Behaviors

- Reward desired behaviors by giving the person something he/she wants or likes, or commenting in a positive way to let him/her know you noticed. Ignore undesirable behaviors.

- Be assertive. This helps prevent conflict and resolve those conflicts that do occur.

- Share your reactions to the behavior. Let the person know when you approve or disapprove, and explain specifically why you feel as you do. In doing this, choose your words carefully so the person does not feel threatened.

- Comment on the behavior rather than the person. Describe what you saw. Do not place blame, make accusations or use name calling.

- Avoid giving advice. Share your ideas and opinions, but don't try to force the person to accept your view. Concentrate on things the person can change. Be positive.

- If your feelings might be a part of the problem or if your actions might be contributing to the problem or behavior, admit it to yourself. Whose problem is it? If the client is cranky, that is his/her problem. If his/her crankiness bothers you, than that is your problem.

- Don't carry around feelings of guilt and blame. If you do, you may become aggressive toward someone else. If you find yourself feeling this way, ask yourself if you are doing all you can to help the client. If you are not, take action once you are doing all you can.

Communicating with Depressed Clients about Difficult Subjects

- Work on building trust. Be friendly and supportive, but not overly cheerful.

- Watch for nonverbal responses to your communication. Sometimes a behavior such as eye contact may be a clue that you're gaining ground. Acknowledge and reinforce any positive response.

- Reinforce your communication with touch. This communicates caring and support.

- If you get no response, leave saying, "I'll be back when you feel better."

- If you make no progress after a period of time, it may be appropriate for another staff member to try and establish a relationship.

- Give the depressed individual space to make choices. Frequently, depression in the elderly occurs following a series of events over which the person had no control such as loss of spouse, loss of home, loss of health or separation from family. Thinking nothing else matters anymore, the individual becomes depressed. Making choices (whether deciding to attend a program or to stay in their room that day) may help the individual feel more in control and less depressed.

- Understand and accept that it is normal to display a variety of emotions including anger and sadness.

- Staff should not shy away from talking about difficult subjects. Being able to talk is one of the most helpful actions a person can take.

- Listen without judging or giving advice.

- Respect the feelings of the person – even if you don't agree with or understand them. Show by your responses that you realize his/her feelings are real and important.

- Develop your personal awareness of natural life occurrences such as aging, loss and death. It is easier to be empathetic with the tough areas others are facing if you have faced these possibilities yourself.

Depression often goes undiagnosed in the elderly. Quite often, if someone has already been diagnosed with dementia, depression symptoms mimic dementia and could easily be misconstrued as a progression of the disease process. Depression is truly the predominate mental illness in the elderly population. For this reason, it is important that you have good communication skills. It's also important to provide meaningful activities that match a client's interests and are modified to their skills and abilities with the goal to enhance self-esteem and reconnect them to who they are as a person.

Providing individualized conversations and activities that recreate positive memories and experiences will both enhance a client's day and increase their quality of life. We must keep the client's psychosocial needs in balance; this can be accomplished through good positive communication. It can be very difficult to communicate with someone who is depressed, because as they decline both physically and cognitively, they utilize behaviors as a means of communicating since words can no longer be used effectively. This difficulty causes both caregivers and family members to feel overwhelmed, and may result in possible premature placement in an assisted living facility or a nursing home.

<u>Overlapping Symptoms of Depression and Dementia</u>

As listed by National Certification Council of Dementia Practitioners (NCCDP)

- Loss of interest in activities
- Appetite changes
- Sleep changes
- Agitation
- Fatigue/lack of energy
- Difficulty concentrating
- Restlessness
- Expressions of worthlessness or guilt
- Repeated thoughts about or talk of death

Non-drug Interventions You Can Do at Home

- Keep a consistent routine. A client's schedule on Monday should be no different than a client's schedule on Saturday.

- Exercise periodically throughout the day (with medical approval). A simple five-minute exercise or walking three times a day is most ideal for a client who is medically cleared to do so.

- Validate feelings. If the client is sad, let them talk about what they are feeling and their thoughts behind the feelings.

- Involve the client in small, meaningful activities throughout the day so that the client can achieve and offer praise for their accomplishments. The use of repetitive activities has been found to be soothing to someone experiencing depression.

- Engage the client in activities they find inspirational and/or spiritual and match their interests.

- The client who is cognitively impaired only has long-term memory. Therefore, all conversations and interactions should be about their past. Create moments of joy.

- Plan a day of beauty.

- Go for a walk. Get outside when the weather is good.

- For more information on the NCCDP, visit www.nccdp.org.

Keys to Communication with Persons who have Alzheimer's Disease

- All individuals with Alzheimer's disease have some difficulty communicating.

- Alzheimer's disease damages the part of the brain that controls communication.

- Memory loss adds to communication problems.

- Individuals may repeat the same word over and over again or use curse words they never used when well.

- Communication is both verbal (22%) and nonverbal (78%).

- Even after they lose the ability to communicate verbally or in writing, Alzheimer's individuals respond to nonverbal communication.

- Keep communication simple. Be calm, speak slowly, and give instructions one step at a time.

- Eliminate distractions and background noise.

- Don't 'talk down' to the individual, and avoid giving commands.

- Don't talk louder if the person does not understand.

- Do not argue. The person is not able to reason and may get upset or angry.

- Validate the other person. Meet the person where they are; join them in their reality rather than trying to convince them otherwise.

- Always look for behaviors, actions or gestures which may convey the feelings or problem the person is trying to express.

- Provide reassurance and comfort. Let the individual know that you care and understand.

Effective Communication for the Impaired Client

"The power and importance of communication is further confirmed by evidence that clients respond to care and live longer when they are engaged in interpersonal relationships with caregivers." (Kely, et. al, 2000)

Verbal Approaches

- Use exact, short, positive phrases. Repeat twice if necessary.

- Speak slowly; give time for the person to answer.

- Use a warm, gentle tone of voice. Talk to them like an adult.

- Only use words that the client is familiar with.

- Give one instruction at a time.

- Make sure you have the person's attention.

Nonverbal Approaches

- Always approach the client from the front before speaking so they can see you and your friendly demeanor.

- Smile and extend your hand to shake their hand. This will communicate that you are friendly and not a threat.

- Get on the same eye level with the person you are talking to – even kneel or sit when speaking to someone.

- Use touch when and where welcomed.

- Identify material items that appear to be important to the client and identify the client's feelings that could be associated with that material item.

    For example: A female client would appear to be obsessing over a handbag and will not do anything unless her handbag is within her sight. The meaning or importance behind the handbag could be that she identifies herself as a woman in control, and women never go anywhere without their handbag.

- Use nonverbal gestures along with words.

- Give nonverbal praise such as a smile and head nods.

Barriers to Communication

There are many barriers to good communication: caregiver barriers, environmental barriers, and medical barriers.

Caregiver Barriers

Caregiver barriers are the primary factor in poor communication.

- Slow down when speaking. Use a calm tone of voice, and be aware of your hand movements.

- Don't raise your voice. Even if not meant in anger, a soft, slow, and calm tone of voice will soothe the client.

- Never demand or command.

- Follow the Golden Rule – You are paid to be wrong all day long. Never argue with a person with an impaired cognition. You will never win the argument.

- Enter their world and live their truth.

- Do not ask memory questions. If the average memory of an impaired client is 20 minutes, asking them what they ate 6 hours earlier or what they did the night before will only make them face the fact that they don't remember and could lead to increased withdrawal and depression.

- Do not offer long explanations when answering questions. Keep your answers to one sentence or even a few words.

Environmental Barriers

Environmental barriers to communication are simply any sounds, conversations or noise competing with your conversation. Environmental barriers include things like:

- Air conditioners, home appliances
- TV
- Outside traffic
- Running water
- Hearing aid batteries that are whistling

Medical Barriers

Medical barriers are barriers you cannot control. However, by being aware of these barriers, you can adjust your communication style. Medical barriers include things like:

- Medication side effects
- Vision impairment or blindness
- Acute illness
- Depression or other mental illness
- Sensory loss
- Pain

Validation: "Living their Truth"

We all have basic feelings and needs as humans. Someone with a cognitive impairment has a diminished ability to communicate with words, and they begin to experience our feelings as well as their own in a very intense manner. The priority when working with clients is best expressed by author Jolene Brackey, who teaches that we should be "Creating Moments of Joy." We should take every opportunity to enter the client's world and experience what they are experiencing – by living in that moment with them. For example, you and your client are looking out the window. You see a parking lot with cars, but your client is talking about the horses outside. This is an opportunity to create a moment of joy. You have two choices: you could say, "There are no horses. What you see is a car in the parking lot." The client would likely respond in an argumentative way since their perception is their own reality. They may even end the conversation and withdraw from sharing their thoughts.

Instead, enter the client's reality while looking out the same window at the same parking lot. The client says, "Wow, look at those horses. They are beautiful." You can respond, "Wow, what kind of horses are they? Tell me about them." Now your client begins to share a memory of when they were younger, and they owned a horse and took riding lessons or won a ribbon at the 4-H fair. If you took the second approach, you would have created a moment of joy by allowing your client to share an important and memorable event in his or her life. It also puts the caregiver in a unique situation because you gained more personal information about that client's passion and past life experience that you can use in future conversations. Your job is to help unlock those cherished memories buried deep in a client's mind.

Many people struggle with the use of validation because it appears as if you are lying to a client or doing a client harm by not keeping them oriented to the truth. You are not lying to the client. You are meeting the client where they are for that specific moment and accepting that this is part of the illness. Feelings are a crucial factor in good communication. When speaking to a client, the caregiver can see emotion from the client, name the emotions, and say, "Jane, you seem angry. What is making you angry?" Always reassure the client. Using validation helps meet the emotional need of a client. The importance of this is discussed in Section I with Maslow's Hierarchy of Needs.

Reality Orientation

Much research has been conducted over the use of Validation vs. Reality orientation. The results overwhelmingly state that there is no benefit to reality orientation for someone who has cognitive impairment. Reality orientation fosters anger, distrust, suspiciousness, grief, and confusion.

Special Approaches for the Aphasic Client

- Get the client's attention before speaking.

- Communicate one idea at a time on an adult level in brief, simple language.

- Speak directly to the client clearly and slowly, yet maintain normal phrasing and intonation. Allow enough time for the aphasic individual to understand what has been said. This may take as long as 10 seconds.

- Combine visual demonstrations with short, verbal phrases when giving instructions.

- Continued repetition of names and commonly used words such as toilet, comb, lipstick, razor or eat is helpful to the client in regaining speech.

- Include the aphasic individual in group activities that do not rely heavily on specific verbal interaction, but which stress social and less demanding interaction.

- Aphasic individuals will normally communicate best when their surroundings are free from distractions.

- A daily routine allows the client to hear the same language and experiences and experience the same situations on a regular basis. Daily routine provides stability and consistency.

- When working with a client, observe any tendency for fatigue, which may contribute to perseveration or catastrophic reactions. Look for signs of stress such as sweating, excessive eye blinking, irritability, and disinterest.

- Don't respond for the hesitant communicator.

- Encourage the client to speak despite any fear or frustration.

- Attempt to communicate with an individual at his/her own level of language functioning – even if it means learning the client's gestural system.

- Talking louder is seldom appropriate.

- Don't be surprised when the client demonstrates inappropriate crying or laughing. This is normal.

- Use of profanity is not unusual and should be taken for granted without penalizing the individual.

- Converse in an unhurried and relaxed manner.

- Don't underestimate the individual's capacity to understand.

- Maintain cheerfulness with the individual while giving emotional support and reassurance.

- Maintain a positive attitude, but be realistic about expectations for progress.

- If verbal communication is difficult for the individual, word all questions in a form that demands only yes/no responses.

Helpful Communication Skills for Visually Impaired Clients

The following tips on communication skills are suggestions and reminders. Given the opportunity, feel free to share these communication skills with the client's family. It may result in a better understanding of the impairment, the client, and his/her specific challenges.

- Identify yourself verbally to the client when you first meet. For partially sighted people, facial recognition is difficult and in many cases, impossible.

- Speak directly and distinctly to the client. Always remember that it is not necessary to talk louder than usual.

- Let the client know when you are about to leave the room or walk away.

- Try to provide specific details and descriptive reference points such as, "The activities room is beyond the office area. You will hear lots of voices and telephones before we get there." Pointing, gesturing or using general statements such as, "It's down the hall," does not give the client enough information.

- Give directions as clearly as possible: left or right according to the direction the client is facing. Sometimes a gentle touch to the arm can be of assistance.

- When showing the client to a chair, place his/her hand on the back.

- Never leave a door ajar. Keep it fully open or fully closed to avoid accidental bumps and falls.

Summary of Effective Communication

Listening allows others to feel noticed and understood. Being a good listener for your seniors requires attentiveness, patience, acceptance, and consideration. Keep in mind some of the following points when interacting with seniors:

Be Attentive

It is not enough to simply listen to a speaker to get what you want. It is also important for the speaker to feel noticed, understood, and taken seriously. Some ways to show your attentiveness include:

- Establishing eye contact with the speaker

- Nodding, or repeating a speaker's point in your own words

- Paying attention to his/her words, gestures, and tone

- Determining what he/she wants from you as a listener. To some, interrupting a conversation to insert your "two cents worth" may be a sign of enthusiasm. To others, it may be a sign of rudeness.

Focus on the Speaker's Story

When a senior begins to tell you about something in their life and you immediately make comments about your own life, you are being a good listener by showing interest in the subject – right? Not really! Though you mean well, you've changed the focus from the senior's story to your own.

There's a difference between contributing to a conversation and taking it over. When a senior brings up a personal or a medical problem, avoid the temptation to tell about someone you know who has a similar problem or worse. By "one-upping" the other speaker, you can make them feel unimportant by stealing their thunder.

It can be natural to take the focus of the conversation away from the speaker, so you may have to work hard to avoid this trap – especially when involved in a conversation with a senior who may have few opportunities to speak. Show interest by asking questions or making comments about his/her story.

<u>Allow the Speaker to Finish</u>

Don't assume you know what the other person wants to say. Avoid the inclination to jump in and finish a speaker's sentence. Sometimes the other person's need to express an idea or a feeling is greater than the information itself. Finishing a sentence may hurt the person who feels you are impatient with him/her. For example, finishing a sentence for a stroke patient may leave the person feeling inadequate as a speaker. The patient might come to the conclusion that he/she is not worth the few extra seconds of your time or that he/she is making you uncomfortable with their speech.

<u>Practice Responsive Listening</u>

Whether the senior in your care is complaining about the food, expressing disappointment about a child's infrequent visits, or rambling on about an imaginary problem, they need affirmation that they are being heard. Respond so that it is clear you are listening and being sensitive to their emotional message. In your own words, repeat the position or complaint as you understand it. Instead of offering unsolicited advice, ask if there is anything you can do to help.

<u>Don't Use Autobiographical Responses</u>

Often we listen autobiographically. People usually respond in one of the four following ways:

1. **Evaluate** – Because of our own history, we sometimes make value judgments about what we hear. A patient may be upset because their child comes only for a short weekly visit. You may also know that while the child is there, the client complains about not staying longer and coming more often. Because of this knowledge, we may inadvertently make a judgment that the client is wrong and the visitor is right. From that point of view, we cannot hear the speaker's pain in their words. Remember, the speaker just needs to know you understand their feelings.

2. **Probe** – We may ask questions from our own viewpoint. For example, if the same client is upset because the child didn't stay the full hour they usually stay, you may find yourself asking questions such as, "Didn't they stay 10 extra minutes on your birthday?" or "How long do you think they should have stayed?" The speaker may not want to deal with more than the disappointment they are already feeling. Although questioning them further may make you feel like you are listening and understanding, they may just need you to share their disappointment and not make them feel that you agree with the child who left early.

3. **Advise** – Do not listen, and then give advice. Remember, your seniors have to work on their own growth and learning.

4. **Interpret** – We often give counsel based on our own experiences and try to explain another person's motives. This approach will not allow the client to make conscious decisions based on their own thought process and evaluation of the event/issue.

Show Empathy

Empathetic listening requires that you validate the client's feelings. You can do this simply by rephrasing the content – affirm in your own words what you think the person has said and reflect those feelings by stating how you perceive the person's feelings. An empathic listener seeks only to understand the speaker's complaint and feelings. An empathic listener does not evaluate, probe, advise or interpret. As a listener, we can empathize with feelings while understanding that sympathy is different and not relevant during the effective listening process.

Make Time for Quality Listening

When a senior begins a conversation at a time when you absolutely cannot listen because you are needed elsewhere, be sure to tell them you can't listen at that time. Reassure them that you would like to hear what they have to say at a different time. Stopping a conversation short or failing to respond at all can be very hurtful. By taking a few seconds to explain your predicament, the other person may feel relieved instead of confused. You may want to set aside extra time to listen to a senior who loves to talk. While an excessive talker may be difficult to endure, they have a psychosocial need for attention that, if ignored, increases the need to be heard even more.

(Excerpts taken from "Powerful Professionalism: The Gift of Listening" by Dee Leone and Becky Daniel, 1998 Gary Grimm & Associates).

Behaviors: What They Mean and How to Deal with Them

Behaviors are nothing more than a means to communicate when words are no longer effective. It is up to the caregiver to uncover the meaning behind the behaviors, and then put a plan into effect to manage those needs.

<u>Repetitive Behaviors</u>

Repetitive behaviors can manifest as repetitive movements, sounds, and words. Typical repetitive behaviors could be repetitive questions, words or phrases; clapping or rubbing of the hands; pacing, often accompanied by a dusting or wiping motion; or rummaging through drawers and closets.

Your job is to uncover the meaning or causes behind the behaviors. First you want to observe for pain or discomfort. Once pain and discomfort are ruled out, the other possible cause could be overstimulation. The section on communication barriers will give you tips on how environmental barriers could be contributing to the overstimulation.

Several interventions are successful when addressing repetitive behaviors. Once it's determined that the movement is not causing harm and the client is not in pain, begin to address both physical and social needs. Address toileting needs as necessary. Create a quiet, calm environment if overstimulation is suspected. You can also distract the client with an activity or conversation. If the client is asking the same question over and over, answer each repeated question as if it is the first time. Be aware of your body language and tone when answering questions. Offer tactile or comfort items as a means to enhance sensory stimulation. This is a great opportunity to incorporate the R.O.S. Legacy System.

<u>Paranoia</u>

Paranoia is the unrealistic belief accompanied by feelings of persecution, blame, and suspicion. If this is a new behavior for your client, and the client has had acute medical illness ruled out as a contributing factor, then look at sensory-related issues. If your client wears glasses and or hearing aids, make sure these appliances are clean and functioning properly. Also pay attention to environmental contributors such as too much stimulation as well as client's basic needs.

Interventions to use for a person who is experiencing paranoia:

- Reassure the client that they are safe, and then begin the validation process. Communicate with the client, find out the details of the situation, and assure them it will be corrected.

- Check glasses and hearing aids.

- Speak in a calm, soft tone of voice.

- Validate their feelings.

- Once the client is calm, investigate to verify or exclude all possibilities.

Aggressive Behaviors

Aggressive behaviors can be defined as hitting, angry outbursts, obscenities, yelling, racial insults, sexual comments, and biting. It can be fearful for a caregiver to communicate or provide care to a client who is aggressive. Just like any other behavior, aggressive behavior is nothing more than a means to communicate what the client can no longer say with words.

Possible Causes for Aggression

- Too much noise/overstimulation

- Cluttered environment

- Uncomfortable temperatures

- Basic needs unmet (toileting, hunger, thirst)

- Pain

- Fear/anxiety

- Confusion

- Communication barriers

- Scared that they do not recognize their surroundings

- Caregiver's mood

- A client perceives that they are being rushed

Using the A-B-C Approach to Behavior Management

(Excerpt taken from www.chicagonow.com/ask-dr-chill/2013/01/managing-difficult-dementia-behaviors-an-a-b-c-approach/)

Managing Difficult Dementia Behaviors: An A-B-C Approach

By Carrie Steckl (a.k.a. Dr. Chill), January 15, 2013 at 3:30 pm

"…In the A-B-C approach, the letter "A" stands for "antecedent," which is a fancy word for something that happens before the behavior in question. The letter "B" stands for the challenging "behavior," while "C" stands for "consequence," or what happens after the behavior occurs.

The idea behind the A-B-C approach is that identifying triggers to a behavior can point us toward ways to reduce that behavior. You've probably heard the joke about the man who goes to the doctor and says, "Doctor, my arm hurts when I move it like this." The doctor replies, "Then don't move it like that!"

The same concept applies here. Most dementia behaviors have a trigger. That trigger might be internal, such as hunger, not feeling well, or having to go the bathroom. The trigger could also be external, such as too much noise, a shower that's too cold or seeing someone or something that frightens the person. If we can identify the trigger, we can try to eliminate it. Doing so might also reduce the behavior.

As caregivers, we also need to pay attention to the consequences of the behavior. Some consequences happen in the environment, such as a fellow grocery patron scowling at you for bringing your loved one to the store. (Do not let this bother you! See my post on reducing stigma for more on this.)

But most consequences to difficult behaviors are our own responses to our family members. When our loved ones become agitated, do we respond in a calm and reassuring way or do we become agitated ourselves? How we respond to a challenging behavior can greatly influence whether the behavior will get worse or better, as well as whether it will happen again.

By using the A-B-C Method, you not only can improve your loved one's well-being, you will experience feelings of self-competence as a caregiver as well."

Interventions to Utilize with Aggressive Client Behaviors

- Communicate for success.

- Reminisce with the client about specific details of their past.

- Validate and support their feelings.

- Identify items they find comfort in, like a picture of the family.

- Provide consistent caregivers and caregiver schedules. Stick to the client's routine.

- Plan recreational activities that match their abilities and interests as tolerated.

- Break down instructions to one-step increments.

- Identify aggression triggers. Be a detective; no behavior just occurs. Keep ongoing communication between family members and caregivers over any noted changes in patterns or behaviors.

- Help the client slow down and relax.

- Play music to calm a person (providing they like music, and ensure if you use music that it matches their interests).

- Use spiritual support if important to the client.

- Remain calm and speak in a soft tone.

Inappropriate Sexual Expressions as a Result of Dementia

Sexuality in the elderly often receives little attention or education. Being aware that inappropriate behavior can manifest itself in a sexual nature will prepare staff to identify and react properly to a client exhibiting these behaviors. Family education also becomes an intricate part of the team approach for a client who experiences these behaviors.

You may see the following behaviors manifest with a person suffering from dementia:

- Behaviors expressed publicly without regard for others
- Touching others sexually without being able to discern if the desire is mutual
- Inability to verbalize 'Yes' or 'No' to sexual advances
- Misinterpreting touches, smiles, and hugs as sexual invitations
- Engaging in sexual acts with someone who is not their spouse or companion
- Disrobing or urinating in inappropriate places
- Sexual comments and/or gestures that might be offensive to others
- Fondling or masturbating in inappropriate places
- Unreasonable jealousy or suspicion

Interventions for Inappropriate Behaviors during Personal Care

- Step back from the client, creating a special barrier.
- Use a calm, firm tone of voice.
- Call the client by their surname to get their attention, creating a formal boundary.
- Identify yourself and your function/intent.
- Do not scold.
- Beware of your body language.
- You may need to excuse yourself from the room. First make sure the client is safe and explain that you will return in a few moments to resume care.

Intervention for Inappropriate Behaviors in Public Areas

- Remove the client from the public area.
- Provide privacy in an appropriate area.
- Provide comfort items as necessary.
- Maintain dignity – no teasing or shaming.

General Interventions

- Observe the client for particular behaviors.
- Check for a possible urinary tract infection.
- Check for genital skin irritations.
- Check for uncomfortable clothing:
    - Too tight or small
    - Too loose
    - Too bulky (if the client is wearing multiple layers of clothing)
- Specialty clothing (clothing dignified by closers located in the back of the garment)
- Model and encourage nonsexual forms of intimacy.
- Offer referrals as necessary for the well spouse.
- Use a fanny pack filled with items to help distract a client who is fondling with clothing below the waist or around genital areas.
    - For women: a fanny pack filled with keys or other items
    - For men: a tool belt

The NDB Model

Need-Driven Dementia-Compromised Behaviors (NDB)

The NDB Model presents a different way of thinking about "problem" behaviors.

- Developed by a group of nurse researchers who sought to better understand and manage "problem" behaviors in dementia
- Arose from the desire to reframe caregivers' thinking and provide an alternative view
- Provides a framework to understand behaviors that have been called:

    ⇒ Difficult

    ⇒ Disturbing

    ⇒ Disruptive

    ⇒ Problematic

ALL Behavior is trying to say something

- Accommodate an unmet need
- Communicate something
- Express a discomfort

The Facts

- Disruptive, agitated, and aggressive behaviors often result from one or more unmet needs – physical, psychological, emotional, or social.
- Loss of ability to express needs in language causes the person to "communicate" through behavior.
- NDB Model emphasizes the interaction between stable, individual characteristics and fluctuating environmental factors that may cause stress or discomfort.
- Assessment is the key to accurate interventions and quality of care.

Essential Features

- Problem behaviors are the result of interaction between:

    ⇒ Relatively stable INDIVIDUAL CHARACTERISTICS

    ⇒ Ever-changing ENVIRONMENTAL TRIGGERS

- Problem behaviors are an "expression" of one or more "unmet needs" – physical, psychological, emotional, or social.
- Persons with dementia are unable to form thoughts or express needs in language.
- Unmet needs emerge in behavior symptoms.
- Comfort and quality of care depend on accurate assessment and intervention.

NDB Behaviors

NDBs take many forms including the following:

- Wandering, elopement
- Disruptive vocalizations
- Agitation and aggression
- Sleep disturbance
- Resistance to personal cares

Management Strategies

- Are highly individualized
- Arise out of assessment data
- Rely on thoughtful review and assessment of:

    INDIVIDUAL CHARACTERISTICS that are fairly stable and longstanding:

    - Health conditions
    - Level of disability due to dementia
    - Personal history and experiences
    - Long-standing personality traits and coping patterns

    ENVIRONMENTAL TRIGGERS that tend to fluctuate and vary:

    - Personal environment
    - Social environment
    - Physical environment

Key to Assessments

Comprehensive and ongoing assessment is vital.

- Describe the behavior: WHO? WHAT? WHEN? WHERE? HOW LONG? HOW OFTEN?
- Ask: Who is this a problem for?

    ⇒ The patient?

    ⇒ Others around him/her?

- Listen carefully for the message the person is attempting to convey.
- Observe for possible "hidden meanings" in actions or words.
- Involve family who may understand the meanings of words or phrases.
- Look for patterns and document habits.
- Attend to nonverbal cues and messages.
- Rule in or rule out medical and/or physical problems.
- Seek to understand the person's internal reality.
- Reframe the problem: Think of the person as FEELING DISTRESSED vs. DISTRESSING YOU.

- Brainstorm with staff and family regarding possible causes and interventions that work even part of the time.
- Reevaluate the situation frequently.

***As a person's status changes due to dementia, so will the response to interventions.

Areas to Assess:

- Overstimulation
- Under stimulation
- Pain/Discomfort
- Immobility
- Psychosis
- Depression
- Fatigue
- Physical design

For full assessment details, see the Iowa Geriatric Education center website, Marianne Smith, PhD, ARNP, BC, Assistant Professor, and University of Iowa College of Nursing.

Five P's of Behavior Management:

1. Define the Problem
2. Learn about the Person
3. Brainstorm possible causes
4. Develop a management Plan
5. Pass it on

Section III

What is "Activities"?

Many definitions of the word *activity* exist including:

- a pursuit in which a person is active
- a form of organized, supervised, and often extracurricular recreation

(*Merriam-Webster's Dictionary*)

The concept of using activities in a medical setting has origins in history as far back as the 1530s. In Greek and Roman times, activities were said to be utilized for combating illness. In the 1700s and 1800s, medical practitioners saw the benefits of using activity for amusement, exercise, and occupational pursuits to treat a variety of conditions. There are records of an asylum in 1830 that used recreational activities and therapeutic games in their medical programs. Even Florence Nightingale gave advice to her nurses in her publication entitled "Notes On Nursing" (1860) which discussed simple ideas on the delivery of activities including:

- "A little needlework, a little writing, a little cleaning would be the greatest relief the sick could have…"
- "Variety of form and brilliance of color in the objects presented to patients are actual means of recovery."
- "Volumes are now written and spoken upon the effect of the mind upon the body."
- "…we must admit that light has quite as real and tangible effects on the human body."
- "Always sit down when a sick person is talking business to you. Show no signs of hurry. Give complete attention and full consideration."

Nightingale went on to discuss the importance of using musical instruments and small pets with patients for both comfort and enjoyment.

In 1929, the first recreation program devoted to studying and providing recreation for handicapped children was established in the state of Illinois. The Veterans Administration added recreation to their programs in 1945 after World War II as a means of distraction to the returning war veterans. By 1960, legislation was beginning to be addressed for specific clients in convalescent centers and rest homes. With the 1987 Omnibus Budget Reconciliation Act (OBRA) which focused on the new regulations, new survey process, and new enforcement procedures, the requirement to employ a qualified activity professional changed the face of activities in long-term care settings and facilities that received federal funding. In turn, these regulations set the groundwork and standards for activities offered throughout health care facilities even today.

Other words/phrases associated with conducting 'activities' with clients could include:

<u>Activity</u> – "all the action and interaction a client experiences during a day" (excerpts from Peckham and Peckham, 1982)

<u>Leisure</u> – "free or unobligated time during which one is not working or performing life-sustaining functions"

<u>Recreation</u> – "activity conducted during one's own leisure" or "a process that restores or recreates the individual…" (Edington, Compton and Hanson, 1980)

<u>Therapeutic Recreation</u> – "…a process which utilizes recreation services for purposive intervention in some physical, emotional, and/or social behavior to bring about a desired change in that behavior and to promote the growth and development of the individual" (Peterson and Gunn, 1984). Or "leisure activity designed to facilitate an improvement and/or maintenance of one's physical and/or mental functioning and/or development growth" (Leitner and Leitner, 1985)

'Activities' refers to any endeavor, other than routine Activities of Daily Living (ADLs), in which a client participates that is intended to enhance their sense of well-being and promote or enhance physical, cognitive, and emotional health. These include, but are not limited to, activities that promote self-esteem, pleasure, comfort, education, creativity, success, and independence. (From the federal regulations for long-term care facilities, F248 interpretive guidelines)

Therapeutic Recreation

Therapeutic recreation programs are a development of functional needs put together by the therapeutic recreation director/specialist, the client, and other individuals who participate in increasing one's lifestyle. Each program has a target which needs to be achieved. Each program should provide creative and comprehensive services to enhance, improve or maintain physical, emotional, mental, social, and spiritual abilities of special needs individuals which could include geriatric, physically or mentally disabled, and chemically dependent individuals.

Programs could effectively address such things as improving physical function and appearance and increasing muscle strength, coordination, flexibility, and mobility. It can build confidence and self-esteem. Therapeutic recreation programs can also promote self-reliance and provide opportunities for creativity, self-expression, self-satisfaction, fun, and self-fulfillment. Some programs could specifically address managing stress, strengthen interpersonal skills, provide opportunities to learn new skills, or enhance skills the client already possesses.

Some types of daily activity that can prove to be therapeutic in nature could include:

Grooming – self-esteem, self-confidence, self-worth, eye-hand coordination, fine motor skills, and independence

Bed making – independence, self-reliance, efficiency, gross motor skills, and coordination

Hand massage – tactile stimulation, interaction, stimulate the muscles/phalanges, and increase blood flow

Board games – provide socialization and interaction skills, improve or maintain cognitive ability, provide eye-hand coordination, and encourage motor skills

Reality orientation – trigger past events, encourage conversation, bring about emotions, and improve eye contact

Activity Services

Activity professionals may provide many of the services mentioned above to their clients within their chosen setting. The extent to which these services are offered depends on the setting and the population within that setting. An activity professional's first priority is to deliver meaningful programs of interest to their clients that focus on physical, social, spiritual, cognitive, and recreational activities.

Activity programs are developed around the information gathered through the assessment process and implemented based on the cognitive ability and individualized functional abilities of the clients that have expressed an interest in that particular program.

Activities by Program Type

Activities are offered through large groups, small groups, and a one-on-one basis, and are developed for individuals with independent interests and abilities to pursue on their own or with minimal assistance. The programs can offer stimulation in either an active form (where the client participates actively) or in a passive form (where the client may sit and listen or observe, rather than actively participate).

Groups

A group setting is the most common setting for most of the programs offered at health care facilities, adult day programs, and senior centers. Group settings allow for socialization and the ability to reach many clients at the same time with the same expressed interest(s). Groups can be divided into three additional sub categories including independent group activities, interdependent group activities or a combination of the two.

Independent groups are those in which each member works as a group, but on individual projects, such as an art class.

Interdependent groups require each member of the group to carry out a specific part of the whole task, such as a cooking group.

In an interdependent/dependent group, members work toward a common goal, such as in a carnival or other event that includes independent and interdependent activities being implemented toward the overall success of the event.

Individual or Independent Activities

Independent activities are typically those activities that a client can do independently or with minimal assistance. They are generally pursued on their own or with some assistance in purchasing materials or setting up the activity. The two types of individual programs include self-directed and individual activity sessions.

In self-directed programs, the client decides to participate in a divisional or hobby activity. This may involve someone purchasing supplies for the client, setting up the room for their activity or even getting additional guidance to complete the task.

Individual activity sessions are those activities in which the client is pursuing things individually such as reading, making phone calls, solving crossword puzzles, crocheting, listening to the radio or sitting in a garden or relaxation room.

Bedside or One-on-One Programs

Bedside programs are appropriate for those clients who are bed bound or who are unable or unwilling to engage in group or independent activity options. A physical illness or cognitive impairment could prevent them from benefitting from any other type of activity engagement. Sensory programs are most appropriate for clients in this situation.

Four factors need to be evaluated when considering bedside activity programs:

1. The person's room and/or environment
2. The client's personal comfort
3. The type of supplies available
4. The timing of the activity

Environment

- Lighting
- Temperature
- Background noises

Personal Comfort

- Position of the client in the bed or chair
- Equipment all in place and working properly such as tubes, pillows, etc.
- Client's ability to hear, see or otherwise manipulate from their position

Supplies and Equipment

- Are the supplies easy to unpack and repack?
- Are the tools prepared so the activity can start promptly without too much prep?
- Can the supplies be put away quickly if the activity needs to end abruptly?

Timing

- Has there been a certain time selected when the client isn't engaged in other ADL activities?

For those in a facility needing bedside visits or one-on-one intervention –

F248 states that one-on-one programming refers to programming provided to clients who will not or cannot effectively plan their own activity pursuits or clients needing specialized or extended programs to enhance their overall daily routine and activity pursuit patterns.

The frequency of one-on-one visits and programs depends on each individual and each one-on-one program. The clients that cannot plan their own leisure generally receive at least three visits each week. The clients that choose not to plan activities can be more of a challenge for regular scheduling, as it would depend on their willingness to participate.

Functional Levels

When planning meaningful activities based on an individual's needs and interests, it's first good to assess the client's functional ability. While there are several definitions of staging levels, for the purposes of this topic we will address the following four functional levels:

Level 1 — The client has good social skills. They are able to communicate their wants and needs verbally. They are alert and oriented to person, place, and time, and they have a long attention span.

Level 2 — The client has fewer social skills and their verbal skills may be impaired as well. The client may have some behavior symptoms or need something to do, and they have an increased energy level with a shorter attention span.

Level 3 — The client has few social skills. Their verbal skills are more impaired than at level two, and they are distracted easily. The client may have some visual/spatial perception and balance concerns, and they need maximum assistance with their care.

Level 4 — This client has a low energy level, nonverbal skills, and they rarely initiate contact with others, although they may respond if given enough time and cues.

Quality of Life

Quality of life is something that we all seek in every age and stage of life. Clients come with their personal history, talents, potential needs, and dreams. The caregiver is one who treasures the history, respects the talents, adapts for the needs, and enables the potential and dreams of each client. Thus, activities are key to providing quality of life experiences for the clients. The interests, strengths, and needs of the client are consistently changing.

Quality of life is different for each person, and it is based on an individual's attitudes and values toward their family, friends, religion, health, work, leisure, environment, lifestyle, etc. Also, an individual's quality of life can change from year to year or from one situation to another, and can continue or change from generation to generational with age. For one person, quality of life might be attending their local church each week and watching television. For another person, their quality of life could include their loved one and eating fruit every morning whenever they wake up. Through the years, those same individuals could be in a different place in life and no longer attend church, but would rather go dancing every week. Quality of life differs for each individual and cannot be dictated by another.

Quality of life can include choices, dignity, and self-determination.

Choices – A client has a right to make independent choices. It is important that a client's individuality and freedom of choice is preserved to the highest extent possible by encouraging them to make personal decisions, such as what to wear and how to spend free time. As caregivers, it is equally important that we make all reasonable accommodations of one's needs and preferences.

Dignity – Recognize a client's individuality by treating the person with respect. The way a client chooses to dress, or the manner in which they choose to style their hair or decorate their environment, the type of religion they choose to participate in, or who they choose to be friends with or love is an individual choice that needs to be treated with respect and dignity.

Self-determination – Self-determination includes the client's right to choose their clothing, meals, and types of engaging, meaningful activity throughout each day. If a client is cognitively unable to make their own choices, then one would solicit advice or input from their loved ones to ensure that their self-directed activity is respected and treated with dignity.

Assessments and Assessment Tools

Assessment

Knowing your client's individual needs, interests, functional abilities, and capacities will assist you in knowing how to plan and engage in meaningful, quality leisure activities.

Definition

An assessment is a systematic process of gathering information about a client in order to make decisions regarding their care and/or their activity program. Assessment is an ongoing process involving the client, family, friends, and significant individuals in the client's life. If the client is in a facility, the assessment team would also be involved in the process. A simpler definition is "the process by which data is collected to identify activity-related resources, strengths, and limitations of the client." Crepeau (1989) states that an assessment is "a narrative process in which initial assumptions are formed…"

In every definition, the details of the individual must be gathered and assessed to provide meaningful opportunities for activities throughout their day and when they are not receiving daily routine activities (ADLs) such as grooming, eating, and resting.

An assessment of the individual should be performed upon the initial meeting with a home care agency, and then periodically thereafter as the needs and interests of individuals are apt to change over time.

Two types of assessments: *Informal* **and** *Formal.*

<u>**Informal assessments**</u> can be utilized to obtain individual background information; past, present and future interests; their lifestyle; personal characteristics; traits; values; what motivates them; and all types of other information that will identify the client's individuality.

Informal assessment tools are implemented through interviews, observation, and information gathered through other means.

<u>Interviews</u> – conducted with either the client or with family members, friends or significant others

<u>Observation</u> – what is seen or observed during the initial meeting phase including what is seen or heard concerning the client, how they interact with others, their behavior, and responses to questions or statements made by others

This observation could take place during the initial contact or through the interview process. Note that initial observations of an individual can change as they relax and become more comfortable with the encounter. Body language and expressions should also be observed during the initial contact and thereafter.

<u>Information gathered through other means</u> – Before a client is admitted to a program such as home health, adult day services, and/or other health care type facilities, a pre-packet of information requesting the client's complete history is required for the facility to assist with getting to know them better.

There are many ways to record this informal information including check lists, fill-in-the-blank forms or via computer, laptop or tablet. The following types of information can be gathered from the client:

<u>Basic information</u> – name, nickname, preferred name to be called, age, DOB

<u>Background information</u> – place of birth, cultural/ethnic background, marital status, children (how many and their names), religion/church, military service, employment, education level, and primary spoken language

<u>Medical and dietary/nutritional information</u> – any formal diagnosis, allergies, and food regimen/diet

<u>Habits</u> – drinking/alcohol, smoking, exercise, and other daily habits

<u>Physical status</u> – abilities/limitations, visual aids, hearing deficits, speech issues, communication, hand dominance, and mobility/gait

<u>Mental status</u> – alertness, cognitive abilities/limitations, and orientation to family, time, place, person, routine, etc.

<u>Social status</u> – social preference, preference for one-on-one interaction, visitation, and communication through written word, phone calls, Skype™ or other means

<u>Emotional status</u> – content, outgoing, introvert, withdrawn, dependent/independent, and emotional abilities and limitations

<u>Leisure status</u> – past, present, and future interests; memberships in clubs; family activities; preferred activity times, and details to individualize client's activities

Formal assessments are utilized to measure specific functional abilities such as physical, cognitive, emotional, and social skills. They are also utilized to assess self-esteem, coping skills, stress levels, interests, and other issues that could pose as barriers to successful participation in leisure activities. The person conducting these standardized assessments needs to be trained to administer, score, and read the assessment correctly. The Mini-Mental State Examination (MMSE), discussed in the psychological aging portion of Section I, is an example of a test to be administered and interpreted by a qualified, licensed physician. An NCCAP certified individual is an example of a qualified person that has been trained to complete a specific assessment tool called the Minimum Data Set (MDS) within a skilled facility to assess the client most effectively in addition to the informal assessment tools.

Formal assessments are standardized, reproducible forms or procedures. This type of format can administer, score and assess/interpret the data collected from the assessment tool. Standardized forms/assessment tools can lend to more comparable data and credibility on the collection of that data.

Standardized assessments must meet three criteria: *Validity, Reliability,* and *Usability.*

<u>Validity</u> – The standardized assessment instrument measures what it is intended to measure. Questions should be relevant and meaningful to garner the most accurate response. Writing questions in a direct format help to obtain and validate data.

<u>Reliability</u> – The assessment tool must accurately examine or measure the stated purpose of the assessment. If the exam is repeated within an established time frame, the results (given the same circumstance) should be the same.

<u>Usability</u> – The chosen assessment tool must be easy to administer and easy to read the results afterwards. The instructions for completion of the tool should be easily understood and include how to score and interpret the scores received through the assessment.

Activity Treatment Potential

A major goal of any successful activity program is the potential for the clients served. Once the client has been interviewed for their interests and their functional ability has been assessed, developing an activity plan can commence. The activity plan can be based on their expressed preference of being with others in a group or being involved in one-on-one activity programs. Depending on the tools necessary to facilitate this request and the number of individuals needed to implement the program, you have everything you need to begin a successful, meaningful activity with your client.

Through the assessment process, you have gathered information about the types of activities you will initiate with your clients. Perhaps they expressed an interest in baking. The goal for the day's activities could be to make cookies with your client. Perhaps they shared their enjoyment of animals. The goal for the day could be to visit the local zoo. Keeping in mind their limitations, if applicable, the focus throughout the activity should be to develop activities giving the clients their maximum potential to work at their highest practical level of functioning whether physically, socially, cognitively, or creatively.

<u>Physically</u> – Rather than maintaining the individual's current level of activity, encourage them to work at their highest level. If exercising, maybe add a few more minutes onto their regimen. If walking, maybe add a few extra steps into the route.

<u>Socially</u> – If the client wants to communicate with their loved ones or friends, rather than dictating a letter to the caregiver, perhaps the client could write their own words or utilize a computer to send an email – even encourage them to Skype™ or utilize other technology to challenge their social abilities.

<u>Cognitively</u> – To encourage a client to work at their highest practical level, they need to be challenged intellectually. If they are solving crossword puzzles, perhaps try harder words. If they are watching game shows, encourage them to respond to the questions prior to hearing the answers. The more a client thinks for themselves, the more they will stay alert and oriented.

<u>Creatively</u> – Once the client chooses the type of creative activity they would like to engage in, such as painting or drawing, encourage them to pick their own colors and use their own techniques. Then give them the tools to augment the best possible outcome.

The preceding scenarios are simple examples of the difference between the client just getting by and the client being encouraged to do the most they can in different areas to enhance their highest potential.

Activities are generally broken down into three different areas – maintenance, supportive, and empowering types of activities.

<u>Maintenance activities</u> – traditional activities that help a client maintain physical, cognitive, social, spiritual, and emotional health

Maintenance activities include:

- Exercise
- Trivia
- Church
- Art classes
- Social clubs

<u>Supportive activities</u> – for clients with a lower tolerance for traditional activities, supportive activities provide a comfortable environment while providing stimulation or solace

Supportive activities include:

- Music
- Meditation
- Relaxation activities
- Massage

<u>Empowering activities</u> – activities that help a client attain self-respect by receiving opportunities for self-expression and responsibility

Empowering activities include:

- Leading the discussion
- Choosing the terms of the activity completely
- Directing a class

Section IV

Importance of Family Involvement in Engaging Activities

Changes in Aging Families

Introduction to Demography of Aging

Demography is the study of populations, their characteristics, and the process by which they change over time. The demography of aging represents the large area of gerontology that can be studied. Social demographers (those people who study the demographics of a population) are generally interested in the age structure of populations and the fertility and mortality patterns that determine how and at what rate populations age.

Demographers also study health transitions, family structure, and marriage rates to better understand the status and well-being of the older adult population. Some questions that they look at regarding aging include: how much ethnic diversity there is likely to be in the future, the number of unmarried elders, and how the longevity and health of the elders are changing over time.

Mortality and Fertility

Almost every nation in the world is becoming progressively older. In just 100 years, the United States has gone from being a nation that consisted of primarily children to one of primarily adults. A couple of factors have led to this transition, including reduced fertility (women bearing fewer babies) and reduced mortality (people living longer). There are four basic transitions in the demographic process determined by the fertility and mortality processes.

Stage 1	The mortality rate for children is high due to poor nutrition and health care. The fertility rate was also higher due to a lack of access to birth control. Additionally, women often had no other role and married and started families quicker than in today's society.
Stage 2	As society modernizes as a result of improved nutrition and expanded health care, infant mortality starts to fall. This fall in infant mortality had an immediate effect on the younger population. Children born during this stage had a much higher chance of surviving.
Stage 3	Fertility rates in a developing society begin to decline due to several factors including less space for bigger families in the urbanization of societies, women fighting for equal rights in the workplace, the delay of marriage and families, and society becoming more prosperous. These changes created a surge in the population of older adults.

Stage 4   The final stage of demographic transition occurs when low fertility rates stabilize for a few generations and the high proportion of older adults also remains stable. Thus the transition to an older society has been completed.

Baby Boomers and Aging in Society

The baby boom represents more than 76 million babies born between 1946 and 1964. The increase in fertility during this time frame has been attributed to the increased prosperity following World War II, which allowed families to have more children since the demand for children was suppressed during The Great Depression and World War II due to tough economic times.

One of the metaphors for this population is "pig-in-the-python," as when a python swallows a pig, it creates a huge bulge as it moves slowly throughout the body of the snake. The baby boomers are doing the same thing in society. Babies meant increased business, increased economy, and an increase in population. Once these baby boomers started retiring around 2007, the population began aging and the economy began slowing down. More than 25% of the workforce today employs individuals over the age of 55.

Baby boomers as a generation do not like to talk about their demise, and in turn are in denial or avoid discussing their long-term plans. Many baby boomers plan to continue working while others are now living in multi-family households, helping to raise grandchildren or continuing to support their middle-aged children. The oldest of the baby boomers are turning 67 in 2013.

Demographic and Social Changes in Families

Population aging caused by declining fertility is manifested at the family level by the elongation of family lineages, meaning more generations (more vertical) and fewer siblings (less wide). As social and historical changes in the structure of families have strongly influenced the functions of intergenerational relationships, it has become more difficult to discuss the family as a single entity as more dynamics are entered into the overall family institution.

Availability of Family Ties in Later Life

The latent kin matrix (Riley, 1983) is a "web of continually shifting linkages that provide the potential for activating and intensifying close kin relationships." An important feature of the latent matrix is that family members may remain dormant sources of support for long periods of time, and only emerge as a resource when the need arises. In more traditional families, the lines of responsibility are more formally drawn, while those in the latent kin matrix tend to respond more voluntarily. This support structure tends to lead the older person to feel uncertain during times of need.

The importance of understanding the family dynamics and each role an individual plays in their family will lend to better understanding and comprehension to that individual's communication and level of engagement in later life with their family, loved ones, and caregivers.

Intergenerational Co-residence

Demographers study family dynamics to determine the number of the elderly population that reside with their children. Older people prefer to live independently of their adult children for as long as possible, however economic crisis in society today has resulted in multigenerational households as a cost-saving strategy.

Three most common reasons cited for living independently:

1. Demographics – Healthy aging implies less need; smaller family size means fewer daughters and fewer opportunities to live with a child.
2. Taste – The cultural preference for living alone reflects values of autonomy and independence in western societies.
3. Economic factors – Increasing affluence of elderly has allowed elders more independence (pensions).

Childless older adults may find communities of age peers appealing with little involvement of younger generations, especially as the adult children become elders themselves. Social change and the aging of the population have resulted in more three- and four-generation families.

Grandparent-Grandchildren Relationships

The growing importance of grandparents –

Only 24% of those born in 1900 were born with all four of their grandparents still alive. Today that number is 68%, which is why grandparents represent a more available resource for the family to rely upon. Single parenting, divorce, and women in the workforce have served to stimulate the involvement of grandparents in everyday life. Such care ranges from babysitting to becoming a full-time guardian for the grandchild when parents are no longer willing or able to fulfill their parenting duties. This changes the involvement from voluntary to fulfilling a fundamental obligation.

Descriptions of grandparenting styles range from surrogate parenthood to being little more than a stranger to their grandchildren. Cherlin and Furstenberg (1985) categorized the relationship styles between grandparents and their grandchildren into the following five types:

1. Detached – little interaction with grandchildren, weak attachment to the role
2. Passive – superficially exposed to grandchildren, but little meaningful interaction
3. Influential – important guide to grandchildren as mentor and advisor
4. Supportive – fun-loving, helps when necessary, offers part-time care
5. Authoritative – quasi-parental figure who disciplines, highly invested in the role

It is most difficult to describe a typical grandparent, as they can range in age from 30 to 100, and their grandchildren can range in age from newborns to retirees. In addition, the role of grandparent is less predictable due to changes in family structure over the past several decades. Grandchildren are also more emotionally attached to their grandparents than previously as a result of becoming the preferred foster care alternative or surrogate parent when a child welfare placement is made by public agencies and court decisions. The prominence of grandparents in the family has grown rapidly.

Marital Relations, Partnerships, and Widowhood

Unpartnered elderly have higher rates of mortality than do married elderly. This mortality rate is evident when the surviving spouse begins to have health problems or suffer their own premature mortality. In other words, close social relationships have the capacity to extend human life. With high divorce rates and lower marriage and remarriage rates, the number of older unpartnered elderly will increase dramatically. Experiencing high-quality relationships throughout life can promote better mental and physical health and lend to longer life expectancy, whereas repeated relationship losses may leave older adults more vulnerable to poorer health, a decline in mental and physical functioning, and perhaps even earlier mortality.

Good relationships can improve health by the following:

- Reducing stress and improving resistance to disease by strengthening the auto-immune system
- Providing practical benefits, such as improved economic security for women (as men were the bigger breadwinners for that generation) and less risky behaviors for men (as they are in committed relationships)

Widow Social Security Benefits

Because of the decline in long marriages, future cohorts may be less likely to qualify for spouse and widow benefits. Fewer divorced retirees will be eligible for spousal benefits based on the 10-year rule applied to marriages. With more women in the workforce, this will make them particularly vulnerable as they will need to rely on their own work records, which often were interrupted by having children or were paid out at a lower rate (initially with women in the workforce).

Changes in Marriage Quality

As marriages occur later, are of shorter duration, and are more likely to be second or even third marriages, it has become a challenge to assess long-term patterns in marriages. The old model used to determine marriage satisfaction (mainly among women) looked at the honeymoon stage as a happier time, then a decline in marriage quality came when having children, yet rebounded once the children grew up and moved away.

A recent review of marriage satisfaction shows a slightly different pattern with men being more satisfied with marriage over the span of the relationship. One of the factors is that men tend to be the benefactors of the work women do in the home such as cleaning, cooking, and child rearing. Another factor could be the fact that parents (mainly women) do not rebound after the children leave home. But rather, they endure empty-nest syndrome and then feel lost over the void in their life. Some give merit to the thought that marriages started in the '50s stay happier than marriages entered into in the '70s. This differentiation in happiness could be due to the changing society or due to the change in the meaning of marriage and expectations that couples bring to their unions over time. The more harmonious marriages are those of older couples or those who waited later in life to marry. After an initial decline, a study by Van Laningham (2001) showed that marriages actually stabilize between 20 and 40 years of marriage and only decline afterward, perhaps as a result of the changing role of spouse to caregiver lending to stress and illness.

Cohabitation

Cohabitation has become much more popular in society today than it was 50 years ago. The stigma involved with cohabitation has changed dramatically over the years, especially with same-sex couples. There is evidence that opposite sex partners are more likely than married partners to end their unions, especially when caregiving becomes evident. Some may argue that opposite sex couples have survived long-term relationships without succumbing to marriage so they may have a weaker commitment to the partnership, while marriage for the most part continues to not be an option for same-sex couples so they may be more vested in the continuance of the union in times of hardship.

Non-Traditional and Alternate Families in Later Life

Step-parenting and Step-grandparenting

Statistically in the United States, one out of every two marriages end in divorce; and most of those who divorce will eventually remarry, causing an impact on multigenerational family life. This rate of divorce and remarriage could also affect establishing long-term ties between parents and their biological children and stepchildren. The role of children and their elderly parents is discussed often, yet the role of the stepchild and their role with an elderly parent or grandparent is one that is not addressed nearly as much.

Gay and Lesbian Families

This is an area that has not been greatly investigated to date, yet will be a focus for understanding how nontraditional families cope with aging in the future, as more nontraditional families are formed in society today. Because to date, same-sex partnerships for the most part do not have legal standings in the majority of states or at the national level, important rights and decisions such as social security survivor benefits are not currently available to same-sex partners. This could have a huge impact on the surviving elder partner if they were not the breadwinner in the relationship and relied on the other partner for their meals, mortgage, and other day-to-day necessities.

Matriarchal Families

This structure is particular common in ethnic minority groups. Single mothers often call on their mothers or grandmothers to serve as a full- or part-time caregiver or surrogate parent for their children. By assisting with childcare, this partnership lends financial support to the single mother who may be faced with economic pressures and may live alone or be close to poverty. When this occurs, a two- or three-generation family is formed where the older women are put in positions of authority over the younger generations within the family unit.

Fictive and Extended Kinship Relationships

These relationships are family-like ties not related by blood, widening the circle of potential family members. This is more common among different ethnic groups, and can change the dynamics of the traditional family by adapting to the changes and, in some cases, energizing the social system. There are more people involved with caring for children or the elderly in this extended family culture.

Childlessness

Childlessness is an area of concern for those who have no children, as they have a more limited pool of individuals to seek assistance from when the need may arise. There are about 20% of childless individuals in the elderly cohort (old-old) in the United States due to more women working longer and unprecedented educational opportunities. Many people have waited to have children, did not have children in their first marriages, and then were too old in the second or third marriage to bear children, thus rendering them childless in their older years. It is estimated that one in four baby boomers will enter old age without children. Being childless is one of the risk factors for being institutionalized. Childless adults will want to plan for alternate family ties or make long-term plans to prepare for old age with little to no support systems in place.

Older Adults as Providers to Family Members

Older adults provide to other generations such things as:

- Child care for grandchildren
- Financial support and bequests to adult children
- Transmitting values to children and grandchildren
- Volunteering to help nonfamily members in other generations

Older people get a lot of satisfaction from engaging in productive and helpful roles, and they may experience improved health and overall well-being, along with a heightened sense of purpose and self-efficacy.

Grandparents as Caregivers

Caregiving grandparents who tend to derive from family, economic, and community context could be themselves challenging and stressful. Such grandparents have to deal with their own issues coupled with those of their children or grandchildren, which could cause them depression or undue stress. There are more than 2.5 million grandparents in the United States alone who are currently raising their grandchildren.

Grandparents as custodial parents can also be beneficial to both the child and to the economy. The term "grand families" was coined to address grandparents as surrogate parents. Typically the grandparents are raising their grandchildren on a voluntary, unpaid basis, which means the older person is contributing to society, yet society is not financially assisting the grandparent in this role.

Caregiving to Adult Children with Disabilities

Older adults support adult children with disabilities who remain dependent for their care and supervision. These can be unique challenges faced by the older adult, especially when their own health or abilities may be diminishing. This challenge might place additional stress on the older person, who may be trying to plan their own long-term arrangements in addition to finding new provisions for their child.

Intergenerational Programming

Opportunities have been developed for older adults to interact with and contribute to the general well-being of younger generations. A blend between seniors and children can be an incredible way to stimulate conversation, improve historical information for the children, and create meaningful opportunities for both generations. Channeling the wisdom, energies, and culture of an older person can only work toward the betterment of the younger generation. Oftentimes, older and younger people are joined in ways that are mutually beneficial to both generations.

Older adults convey important values, attitudes, and beliefs to younger generations while providing them with the cultural capital necessary to become well-functioning adults. Children, in turn, offer the older adult diversion, unconditional love, respect, and an avenue to feel an intricate part of society.

Caregiving for Older Relatives

Family caregiving as informal long-term care

Caregiving is defined as "help and support provided to chronically impaired individuals" that may need help or assistance or may have difficulties with an activity of daily living (ADL) or instrumental activities of daily living (IADL).

ADL – personal tasks such as bathing, toileting, and dressing

IADL – goal-oriented tasks such as housework, cooking, laundry, and shopping

Incidentally, the area not referenced in the terminology of caregiving and the support that caregivers can provide is the very subject this document addresses: the benefit of engaging an individual in meaningful activities outside of ADLs.

Caregiver Facts:

- 2/3 of caregivers are women (wives and daughters).

- Daughters tend to provide hands-on, health-related care giving, while sons typically assist with transportation.

- 3/4 of caregivers hold full-time jobs while tending to the needs of the elderly individual, which could lend to the need to switch work schedules, reduce work hours or quit their own jobs to tend to the needs of others.

- The majority of caregivers are over the age of 50.

- Caregiving tends to be devalued in society today – not considered economically productive and, in turn, does not receive medical benefits or accrue retirement hours.

Caregiving and Gender

Women are the primary source of social support and care for older people. With the ratio of men to women being approximately one male to eight women, it comes as no surprise that women are predominantly the caregivers. Men rely on their wives while women tend to rely on family members for their physical needs once they are widowed.

Daughters are often more likely to provide care for their older parent(s) than any sons. One reason may be that the societal gender role has directed girls to perform more of the hands-on care, while boys perform more of the outside work such as yard work and car repairs. As the stereotypical roles of males and females change, a shift will also take place with caregiving practices.

A more feminist perspective could be that women have often been channeled into the lower paying, less appealing jobs. Caregiving, by nature, is not typically a high-paying job or one with much clout, and so it would be a woman's job, rather than that of a man – free labor if you will. The shift in society since the mid-1970s has altered this job burden and will continue to adjust as societal norms change with the times.

Caregiver Stress

Several factors can contribute to caregiver stress:

- Time management difficulties

- Fatigue and physical strain

- Work/family conflicts

- Conflict with other family members over who will provide care, financial support, etc., when needed

- Lack of time to take care of one's own needs

- Financial worries over the cost of caring for a loved one

- Potential isolation - being cut off from one's own friends and activities as a result of committing so much time to caring for others

Stress can lead to: exhaustion, high blood pressure, depression, anxiety, and other physical ailments and psychological distress.

The Caregiver Stress Model

Excessive caregiving (burden) induces stress, which in turn elevates levels of distress.

Caregiving burden – problems managing the tasks of caregiving

Stress – appraisal of caregiving as causing strain or other physiological stressors

Distress – poor emotional or physical well-being

Coping – managing burden and stress by mobilizing resources and making the necessary cognitive adjustments

Coping skills can alleviate the feelings of burden and distress by lowering the reaction to both. Problem solving is one of the most effective methods to alleviating that stress. Getting outside help and taking time off is more proactive then avoiding the issues or denying the problems associated with caregiving.

Social support is another coping mechanism that can break the monotony and avoid negative experiences. There are several formal programs available for caregivers aimed at lowering stress and burden, such as respite programs, counseling, and exercise programs to relieve stress. There is no reason for a caregiver to go through the process alone when it is much more manageable with support.

National Family Caregivers Support Program (NFCSP)

In 2000, the Older Americans Act was amended to include the NFCSP, developed to include the informal caregiver as a target client within the old age program. The NFCSP recognizes that the older person often receives care from family members and friends who themselves may need support to continue their efforts. This program spends more than $150 million a year and allows states to provide a continuum of services to adults of any age and income level who care for impaired individuals at least 60 years of age. It includes the following:

- Assistance to caregivers in gaining access to services
- Information to caregivers about available services
- Individual counseling, organization of support groups, and caregiver training
- Respite care

Family and Medical Leave Act (FMLA)

The FMLA Act guarantees 12 weeks of unpaid leave to caregivers without the threat of losing their job. The worker is protected during this time off in order to return to their job after taking the leave of absence. There are, however, some exemptions for small businesses, which can often allow for no guaranteed leave.

Variation in Support of Old Age in Different Countries

In the last several years, studies have been conducted to understand the importance of caregiving practices across different cultures and societies. The economies, political systems, family patterns, demographic structures, and cultural values of different societies form a backdrop to the organization of care and support for older individuals and the role older individuals play in their families. China, for example, differs from the United States as more than 69% of their elderly reside with their children compared to 20%, as a result of the filial responsibilities practiced.

Families differ from each other in many ways. The family dynamics, level of involvement, and types of interactions between family members can hurt or enhance the quality of life for their loved one, family member or friend. One thing is consistent, involved families make a difference. They can support, encourage, and uplift those in their care by engaging clients and providing meaningful activities throughout the day.

Section V

How to Engage Clients

Caregivers and activity professionals play a therapeutic role in each client's health care management. In a broader spectrum of health care, the work performed by caregivers can often be perceived as fun and games or just keeping someone busy. In actuality, providing therapeutic, meaningful, and engaging activities can help minimize the risk of boredom, depression, and behavior problems. So, how can professionals engage someone to participate in activities?

As humans, we all have a need to be productive and purposeful. As the family member or caregiver, you must discover a senior's motivation, then give the senior a reason (that makes sense to him/her) to participate and be active.

When engaging someone in activities, keep these goals in mind:

- Prevent withdrawal or deterioration

  - Treat the client as an individual. Ensure that activities and conversations are relevant to the client and his/her life.
  - Incorporate parallel programming in group settings. Divide participants by functional abilities; each sub group will participate in the same activity at individual levels of independence.
  - Seat people of like cognition (intellectual level) together. This will help the facilitator manage the activity and quickly offer assistance as needed.
  - Adapt the activity through planning and preparation. Focus on a client's abilities, and then modify the activity to allow participation at the highest practicable ability.

- Train or re-train recognition of articles once familiar

  - Print a variety of simple pictures to use as flash cards. Show the client a picture. If he/she has trouble naming the objects, offer one clue at a time until the client correctly identifies the object.
  - Montessori-Based Dementia Programming (MBDP) is a method of working with older adults living with cognitive and/or physical impairments. Based on the ideas of educator Maria Montessori, MBDP has been shown to increase levels of engagement and participation in the activities of persons with dementia. While MBDP cannot cure or prevent Alzheimer's disease, it has been shown to generally improve many quality of life aspects.

- Montessori-Based Dementia Programming uses rehabilitation principles including guided repetition, task breakdown, and progressing from the simple to complex.

- Utilize physical and mental capabilities

    - The World Health Organization states that (with medical approval) seniors should exercise at least 45 minutes throughout a day, not all at once.
    - In adults aged 65 years and above, physical activity includes leisure time and other activities such as walking, dancing, gardening, hiking, and swimming; transportation (e.g., walking or cycling); occupational activity (if the individual is still engaged in work); household chores; play games, sports or other planned exercise in the context of daily, family, and community activities.
    - Exercise will improve cardiorespiratory and muscular fitness, bone and functional health, and reduce the risk of depression and cognitive decline.

- Accept present surroundings

    - Validation - The basic principle of validation therapy is the concept of validation or the reciprocated communication of respect, which communicates that the opinions of others are acknowledged, respected, and heard. Regardless of the listener's level of agreement, the speaker should always be treated with genuine respect as a legitimate expression of their feelings, rather than being marginalized or dismissed.

- Maintain or stimulate interests and social contacts

    - Once the family completes the personal history and interest assessment, begin to utilize that information to build a daily routine and incorporate activities that specifically match the client's interests and abilities. This approach will provide personal information that the client can talk about.

- Focus on human worth

    - Providing activities that clients can succeed at will increase their self-esteem. We all have things in our lives that make us proud or give us passion – things that define a person as a productive member of society and allow them to discuss what they are passionate about. Generally speaking, people like to talk about themselves and what is important to them.

    - It can be surprising to engage a client in an activity meant to enhance their cognition, such as a trivia game or a wordsearch puzzle, that results in 30 minutes hearing stories never heard before or having been heard a million times. For the client, you have unlocked a passion. Though the details may have changed over the years, this is a special moment that you created for your client.

- Distract away from physical condition

    - It can be quite discouraging to always be reminded of physical limitations and what you can't do. Instead of focusing on disabilities, create an environment that enables your client to participate at his/her own level and pace.
    - You may have a client who can no longer go deep-sea fishing, but you can utilize fishing rods, wicker baskets, hats, lures with hooks removed, and enlarged pictures of past fishing experiences to reconnect that person to his/her interests and passions.
    - It can be easy to think that reminding clients of activities they can no longer do will upset them; however, research and case studies show that the opposite is true.

Case Study:

There was a 37-year-old male nursing home resident who had been in a motorcycle accident which left him a quadriplegic. After two years in an acute rehabilitation hospital, he came to live in a nursing home. A new activity director was hired 18 months after the man was admitted. During her assessment of the resident we will call "Scott," he presented as having the ability to move his head and focus his attention on who was speaking to him. Scott grunted, but did not display this as an ability to communicate. His mom visited often, and was very defensive when a personal history was presented. She did not see the value in a personal history and provided very limited information.

The activity director charged with creating an individualized activity program started with a consultation from the physical therapist and occupational therapist. The activity director wanted proper seating position equipment as well as adaptive equipment that would focus on his abilities and allow him the ability for leisure enjoyment. The first activity was a painting activity. Scott received a wheelchair with advanced pressure-relieving cushions and a tabletop easel so materials could be positioned for him at eye level. Scott was then fitted for a head pointer with an attached paintbrush.

The day came when the staff would see if their efforts would be successful in creating a positive environment and adapting an activity to allow the client to be as independent as possible and function at his highest practicable ability. The staff explained to Scott that he was going to paint on canvas. They attached the head pointer and paintbrush, dipped the brush in paint and positioned the paintbrush on his canvas. He began to move his head, which moved the paintbrush and applied paint to the canvas. After a few moments, Scott had finished his abstract artwork and he lowered his head. We wondered if he was done or perhaps this was a way to signal staff that this work of art was completed.

The staff changed the paint color and gave Scott a new canvas. Scott lifted his head and began to paint again. That day, Scott independently painted four pieces of art that were proudly displayed in his room. Several days later, his mom came and saw the artwork. Her initial response was anger, then sadness. The activity director met with her, and through the tears she explained that prior to Scott's motorcycle accident, he was an avid painter. The doctors at the hospital were convincing her to not put him on life support and said that her son would be a "vegetable." They said he would be unable to do anything ever again. She thought she was acting in his best interests by not sharing his past passion of art because she thought she was protecting him from remembering what he no longer had the ability to do. That day, Scott was able to paint for his mother.

Painting had a profound impact on Scott's life from that moment forward. In the years that followed, Scott woke every day and began communicating with head nods. The facility hosted an art show for him and people came from across the state to meet Scott and purchase his art. From that day forward, the activity director promised to never look at someone and make an assumption of what they can or cannot do. The staff would use each person's abilities and adapt their environment so they can both enjoy and engage in their favorite activity and live the best quality of life imaginable.

- Alleviate distress

  - Maintain a consistent routine. Be consistent in your approach and your answers.
  - When multiple caregivers, staff, and family members provide care and assistance to a client, develop a communication book to document the person's daily routine. Note approaches that are successful when trying to motivate the client. If the client tends to ask the same question repeatedly, ensure that family members and caregivers answer consistently.
  - For example, if the client asks, "Where is Mabel?" it is important to know who Mabel is and what her relationship is to the client. Then provide an answer that makes sense. If Mabel is the client's daughter and the client thinks Mabel is eight years old, a typical eight-year-old would be in school during the day. The challenge comes when one person responds that Mabel is in school and another person responds that Mabel is at work. This disparity in answers could cause more stress for the client. The client could become agitated: if no one knows where Mabel is, then she must be lost and needs to be found. Or if Mabel is at work, is she alright? Wrong answers or answers that don't make sense cause more stress, which in turn triggers behaviors that could be more difficult to manage.

- Provide an outlet for irritation

  - Client Support: Many support groups exist for clients who are facing personal, physical, and emotional loss.
  - Caregiver and Family Support: Many local support groups are free to caregivers and family members. Stress can cause the caregiver or family member a number of health-related issues, and caring for oneself is equally as important as caring for clients. Families and caregivers are encouraged to know their limits and get the support they need.
  - Encourage family members to maintain their role as family and allow the caregiver to do their job. This encouragement will help alleviate any feelings of guilt or abandonment that the family member has failed their loved one by calling 'strangers' to care for the family member.

- Promote speech

    - Always encourage clients to talk, share stories, and communicate. Clients with dementia may start to present with difficulties finding the right words. If still cognitively aware, these losses could make the individual become frustrated and cause them to avoid talking altogether.
    - Avoid trying to finish sentences or correcting them if they are wrong.
    - Review the communication section for tips and suggestions on verbal and nonverbal communication.

- Promote controlled fatigue

    - Controlling fatigue is an important part of building an activity plan. If someone has had a good night's sleep and is still sleeping throughout the day, the client could be over or under stimulated. The caregiver should balance the stimulation to control fatigue. The client should be active as tolerated but, when it is time for bed, it is most beneficial when the client is exhausted and sleeps through the night. Engage the client in structured daily activities that are short in duration so that at the end of the night, they are tired and ready for bed.

Best Practices for Engaging Clients with Dementia

- Complete a Personal History Interview

    - We have provided examples of basic and key information for a caregiver or other health care agent to know about a person.
    - The family member(s) should be asked to complete the Personal History Form along with the Interest Page in Section VIII. The family may need a few days to allow for appropriate time to thoroughly complete the information. Encourage the family to involve all family members and close friends in completing this information. This Personal History Form should be shared with caregivers who enter the home and should follow the client through the spectrum of health care settings.

- Activities are person appropriate

    - Centers for Medicare and Medicaid Services (CMS) defines *person appropriate* as the idea that each resident has a personal identity and history that includes much more than just their medical illnesses or functional impairments, and that activities should be relevant – as much as possible – to the specific needs, interests, culture, background, etc., of the individual for whom they are developed.
    - Person appropriate will be discussed in detail in the next section.

- Redefine your idea of an activity program

    - Active activities can include baking, basketball, beanbag toss, sing-a-longs, crafts, clipping coupons, dancing, holiday decorating, folding clothes, safe and appropriate light domestic chores, letter writing, nature walks, rolling yarn, sanding wood, and sorting objects.
    - Passive activities can include arranging flowers, listening to bible stories, blowing bubbles, making collages, solving crossword puzzles, solving wordsearch puzzles, reading devotions, looking at magazines, applying lotion to hands, listening to music, reading poetry, smelling herbs and spices, participating in a spelling bee, watching TV, or reminiscing about stories.
    - Memory boxes, theme-based containers that include a variety of props and pictures related to a certain theme, can be a great way to help keep clients connected to their past. Have family members help create a theme box from materials in their home based on the client's interests and passions. Examples for themed boxes include:

- Art Box – contains paintbrushes, canvas boards, finished paintings or drawings, and colored pencils.

  Ask the client to identify these items and their uses.

- Baby Box – contains baby clothes, baby dolls, diapers, baby booties, stuffed animals, lotion, music box, and a baby blanket.

  The experiences that affect someone over their lifetime can include dating, attending weddings, having children, gaining an education, holding a job, managing a career, and focusing on family life. Therefore, the baby box described above is just one example of a life experience box that can be created for the client.

- Jewelry Box – can contain costume jewelry, as clients and family members may be concerned about having family heirlooms and valuables accessible to others.

- Reminiscing Box – contains specific items that are mementoes of the person including pictures and other collectables they have treasured throughout their life.

Things to Remember

As the disease progresses, parts of the brain die along with the memories and abilities controlled by that part of the brain, so an 80-year-old woman's brain may only hold the memories and abilities of a seven-year-old girl.

Engaging Activities for Someone with Difficult Behaviors

- Reduce Noise and Visual Distractions

  - Limit group size, limit the number of people giving instructions, limit distracting background noise (TV, radio, etc.)
  - Make sure you have the client's attention when speaking.

- Increase Environmental Cues

    • Ensure the client has proper lighting for the activity.
    • If eating is a problem, then only use the kitchen table for eating and find another place in their home to engage in other activities. The same concept can be applied to lying in bed and watching TV. The bed and bedroom should be utilized for sleep. Keeping distinct areas in the house used for the sole intended purpose will help provide boundaries and reduce difficult behaviors.

- Maintain Schedules

    • Maintain each client's normal schedule as much as possible. Keeping a consistent schedule with daily routines will provide the client a sense of security. A weekday should look the same as a weekend.

Suggested Program Approaches for Clients Who Exhibit Difficult Behaviors

1. **Problem of Concern:**
   - Client is experiencing episodes of paranoia that hinder their daily activities and seem to cause stress.

   Approaches and Intervention (that may address or eliminate the concern)

   - Offer topics of discussion based on their past leisure experiences and interests.
   - Keep daily routines consistent.
   - Reinforce reality focus.

2. **Problem of Concern:**
   - Client is not showing safety awareness, evidenced by putting foreign objects in their mouth.
   - Client grabs or pinches others or rocks their upper body.
   - Client appears anxious and presents with wringing of hands, rigid posture, pacing or jumping at every sound.

   Approaches and Intervention (that may address or eliminate the concern)

   - Determine and eliminate the trigger. A violent TV program? Too much noise?
   - Offer activities that are repetitive in motion such as coloring or sorting and folding clothes.

- Repetitive movements have been shown to deescalate behaviors.
- Only use nontoxic materials that do not pose a choking hazard. Rule of thumb: use nothing smaller than your elbow.
- Focus the client's attention on emotionally soothing activities such as listening to music and talking about their strengths and skills. Give much sincere praise.
- Ask the client direct, open-minded questions to promote conversation.

3. **Problem of Concern:**
   - Client expresses feelings of sadness.
   - Client appears to be irritable, evidenced by scowling when approached or answering questions in a curt, unpleasant manner.
   - Client seems to be withdrawn from previously enjoyed activities or displays worried facial expressions or a slumped posture.

   Approaches and Intervention (that may address or eliminate the concern)

   - Remind client of the pleasant aspects of the activity they previously enjoyed.
   - Offer frequent positive reinforcement for any displayed level of involvement.
   - Model a relaxed demeanor, as emotions can be mirrored.
   - Help the client identify positive traits about themselves.
   - Engage in activities that give the client a sense of value. Refer to his/her Personal History Form.

4. **Problem of Concern:**

   Client at times is disruptive, becomes demanding, cries uncontrollably or becomes uncontrollably angry.

   Approaches and Intervention (that may address or eliminate the concern)

   - Repeat activities proven to be successful. Completing the evaluation section of the activity lesson plan will serve as a communication tool.
   - Involve the client in familiar, work-related activities.
   - Stop the activity if the client becomes tense, preventing the client from becoming overwhelmed.
   - Involve the client in physical activities to burn energy.
   - Give instructions one step at a time.
   - Provide activities that are repetitive in nature.

5. Problem of Concern:

Client presents with aggressive outbursts such as threating family or caregiver, or episodes of shoving, hitting, and scratching.

Approaches and Intervention (that may address or eliminate the concern)

- Make sure client's basic needs are met for his/her comfort. Review Maslow's Hierarchy of Needs for more explanation.
- Present all communication and movements in an unhurried pace.
- Use listening skills to identify the source of aggression.
- Remind the client of the necessity to not hit or threaten others.
- Offer activities that match interests and are broken into smaller steps so the client can succeed and accomplish goals.
- Try activities that are repetitive and can be stopped if the client becomes overwhelmed.

Programming for Individuals with Mild to Moderate Dementia

Many clients have cognitive deficits that are significant enough to impact their day as well as awareness of their surroundings. By providing activities that reinforce their past, we increase and improve their social skills which then improve their general interactions with others. When a client is disoriented, validation activities are successful because their focus is emotions and feelings. A caregiver can also utilize remotivation or reminiscing activities which are appropriate for the client who is aware of self and seeks out others to engage in socialization. Finally, caregivers can use resocialization activities for clients who have intact socialization skills and would benefit from activities geared toward maintaining an awareness of person, time, and place.

<u>Validating Activities</u>

- Validating activities authenticate the memories and feelings of individuals who are very disoriented. They focus on a client's perception of what happened in the past. Naomi Feil, founder of validation methods, suggests not to focus on orientation, but rather a person's perception of what happened in their past.

- Clients who exhibit these characteristics would benefit from validating activities:
    - Someone who has moderate disorientation, such as time or place confusion
    - Someone who is unaware of their environment and may make repeated statements such as, "I need to get home," even though they may be in their home
    - Someone who lacks rational thinking, such as turning on the oven to heat the house or using a knife instead of a fork
    - Someone who is easily distracted and needs to be redirected in thought or during a task

- Making validating activities work (an excellent method when dealing with someone with aggressive behaviors):

    - Use touch when welcomed. You will know which clients enjoy having you rub their back, hold their hand or touch their knee. When someone welcomes touch, this can be a great nonverbal sign of safety, security, and love.
    - Maintain eye contact and be aware or nonverbal communicating styles.
    - Remember, emotions will be mirrored.

- Be clear with your words. Use words that are familiar to the client, and speak slowly in an unhurried pace.
- Acknowledge and name the feelings that the client may be displaying.
- Validate that the client looks worried, then ask the client to tell you why they are worried. Use active listening skills for meanings behind the spoken word.

- Validate verbally both feelings and fantasy:
  - Ask if he/she needs to go home and feed the children.
  - Acknowledge thoughts.
  - Acknowledge experiences as a parent.
  - State or affirm something nice about his/her children.
  - Unravel the meaning behind responses and body language during conversation.

Reminiscing Activities

- These activities are designed to help the client see that they have contributed to society by looking at their past achievements. In the client's development, it is important to see oneself as a contributing member of society.

- Remotivational activities include, but are not limited to:
  - Allowing the client to see themselves as part of the community, not just as an individual
  - Engaging the client in thinking about the world and world events as they are today
  - Increasing the sense of reality with the client

- Reminiscing activities can be utilized for people who are:
  - Displaying fearful actions and/or have decreased cognition, evidenced by short-term memory loss or forgetfulness
  - Passive and enjoy being an observer, rather than an active participant
  - Able to follow directions – even if those directions need to be broken into smaller steps

To ensure these type of activities are successful you must guarantee:

- Consistency with approach, schedule, and communication. Consistency across the spectrum of care environment is essential.

- Use clear, concise communication both through verbal and nonverbal styles.

- Give constant praise and encouragement. Individuals, by nature, are people pleasers. They want to please their parents, supervisors, teachers, and themselves. By providing praise and encouragement, you will see an increase in participation and effort. This includes giving immediate feedback for involvement and praise. At this phase, the client may need immediate gratification and acknowledgment of their efforts.

- As with praise and encouragement, you want to reinforce the client's strengths and abilities while also reinforcing their individuality, life achievement, and contributions.

- The use of appropriate humor and sincerity of ebbing yourself is also an important factor to making these activities work. It is okay to share personal stores with the client. It will help them relate to you as more than a caregiver and will also allow for sharing common experiences.

Once you have reminisced, you begin to remotivate, and that leads to resocialization.

Resocializing Activities

- Once a client can successfully participate in reminiscing and remotivation activities, it is time to encourage them to build on those social skills and begin to expand their connections to the community. Reconnecting can be as simple as communicating with a neighbor or participating in church or within the community.

- These activities also allow the client to explore their feelings and turn those feelings into meaningful interactions.

- Goals of Resocializing Activities:
    - Complete the transition and engage the client in the community.
    - Assist the client in identifying the benefits of finding interest in other activities. Remind the client of the importance of involvement, civic duty and the feelings they experienced by being part of something bigger than themselves. Involvement will help your client promote a greater sense of independence and increase their self-esteem.
    - Build the client's social skills by increasing their ease in social encounters with others.

Challenges of Talking to Someone with Alzheimer's or Other Related Dementias

In Sections I and II, we talked about the decline and challenges a client may face if they have Alzheimer's or other dementias. Engaging these clients is often difficult because of their short-term memory loss and heightened expression of feelings. Prior to the client's illness, one would engage in a normal conversational routine of "How are you?", "What did you do today?", "What's new with you?", and other such routine statements. However, questions rely on short-term memory, which is lacking in the Alzheimer's client. Here are some strategies as recommended by the National Alzheimer's Association:

Topics Guaranteed to Get Discussion Started with Seniors with Dementia

- Colors
- Surprise bag
- Fashion show
- Favorite music
- War stories
- Holidays
- Home cooking
- Sports
- School days
- Old cars
- Information included on Personal History Form

What to Say/Do When There's Nothing to Say/Do

- Say, "I love you," "I came to see you," or "I'll be back again," (regardless of their reaction to your visit)

- Sit close, away from window glare, and at eye level, then touch or hold as preferred by the client.

- Look for clues of feelings through body language, eyes, or repeated phrases.

- Gentle teasing or joking provides a sense of continuity and pleasure to those who have always communicated this way in their families.

- Silence can be golden – tender moments watching birds, listening to music or praying can be wonderful for both client and caregiver.

- Respect personal space and possessions. Ask before moving things around or sitting on the bed. Go slowly and keep pace with the person's concentration, tolerance, etc.

- Substitute shared activities for those with limited conversation: manicures, massages, looking at photo albums, watching TV, walks, writing letters, etc.

- Reminisce about your favorite holiday, first car, baking in the old home, the smell of a wood fire. Note: If the client is very impaired, talk about earlier events.

- Use the arts and your skills such as music, poetry, photos, video, audiotapes or artwork to stimulate the person. Play games. (Even if the client can't play as well, they may still enjoy the activity.)

Programming for Individuals with Severe Cognitive Impairments

Severe cognitive impairment might best be defined as someone who has little ability to care for their most basic needs. When working with clients, strive to stimulate a person's response and promote the highest level of abilities. Break down tasks and simplify instructions as the client's skills diminish. These clients may be unable to plan their own day, but they have not lost interest in being entertained.

There are two specific types of interventions that can address the person with severe cognitive impairment: Sensory Integration and Sensory Awareness / Sensory Stimulation.

Sensory Integration

- The caregiver or family provides basic stimulation of the client's senses: seeing, hearing, body awareness, balance, and touch.

- This program is utilized for individuals who are in later stages of Alzheimer's or dementia.

- Activity Goals for Sensory Integration:

    - Improve the cognitive physical, emotional, and functional abilities of the individual.
    - Increase a client's attention span, which can be very limited for the client with severe cognitive impairment. This focus will also increase the capacity for interactions and the tolerance level of social and physical interactions.
    - Promote fine motor and gross motor skills by encouraging the use of fingers and hands.

- Examples of Sensory Integration Activities:

    - Encourage movement of the head.
    - Design activities that encourage the use of fingers and hands, which allow the brain to open up to new information. Examples: clapping hands, using hand puppets, playing string games, pulling taffy, painting, window wiping, hand holding, hand massages, and manipulating materials that have a hook-and-loop closure.
    - Incorporate tactile discrimination, manipulating items with different textures such as sandpaper, soft and hard textures, or cold and warm textures.
    - Craft activities which provide body awareness experiences such as the use of makeup brushes to brush across face or placing marbles in a shoe box filled with sand and running hands through the sand.
    - Create art with paint rollers; this activity moves the left arm across to the right and vice versa, which crosses the midline of the brain hemispheres so the client develops a greater repertoire of responsiveness.

Sensory Awareness / Sensory Stimulation

- Provides various types of stimulation with the express purpose of eliciting a response from the individual

- Reactions may or may not be logical responses to the types of stimulation provided

- The strongest sense is our first sense – the sense of smell

Sensory Stimulation Activities

Sensory stimulation activities are used to help clients increase their interaction with the world around them and are intended to elicit a meaningful response to the stimulus.

- Sight/Vision – hidden objects, colorful objects, slides, tracking activities, electronic games, electronic tablets, maps, mirroring, posters, photos, and flashlights

- Touch/Tactile – Fingers are filled with multiple receptors that are stimulated by shapes and textures. The lips are also very sensitive to touch. The skin is the largest sensory organ of the body. REMEMBER to use touch only when it is welcomed. Respect personal space. Place objects in a box or in sand and have the client hold the object without seeing it and try to describe what he/she is holding. Make it a theme ... provide clues.

- Taste – Have the client close his/her eyes and place different foods in their mouth, then have them identify the taste. Use foods and flavors such as pickles, maple syrup, oranges, vanilla, nutmeg, lemon, peanut butter, and peppermint. BE AWARE of diet restrictions and allergies.

- Smell/Olfactory – Stimulate the sense of smell by using vinegar, nutmeg, apple, vanilla, coffee, lemon, lavender, and cloves. (BE AWARE: Cloves are poisonous if ingested or used as a pain killer.)

- Hearing/Auditory – Try pouring water into a container, rubbing wood against wood, shaking a wind chime, clinking ice in a glass, jiggling coins together, and other common environmental sounds.

The goal is to continually simplify tasks so they remain within the client's diminished abilities, allowing them to retain as much control over their life as possible and to maintain personal dignity. Simplifying tasks could decrease negative behaviors as well as the use of restraints.

Sensory stimulation programming is for people who are experiencing decreased judgments and initiative, and are unable to recognize familiar objects.

Baby Boomers

Baby Boomers are people born between 1946 and 1964. During this period of time, the United States saw an explosion in birthrates that had never been seen before, and nothing like it has been seen since. Today, baby boomers make up approximately 28% of the total U.S. population.

With this group of people occupying such a large segment of the population, it is predicted that there will be a major financial strain on the health care industry as baby boomers reach retirement age. There are many reasons why the health care industry will face problems as baby boomers begin to retire and need more health care services.

As a group, baby boomers were the wealthiest, most active, and most physically fit generation up to that time, and amongst the first to grow up genuinely expecting the world to improve with time. They were also the generation that received peak levels of income; therefore they could reap the benefits of abundant levels of food, apparel, retirement programs, and sometimes even midlife crisis products, such as sport cars, boats, or other status items.

Understanding the demands of the baby boomer generation and preparing for their psychological needs now will help as more and more baby boomers retire and may be in need of additional health care services.

Psychosocial Needs of Baby Boomers

www.ltlmagazine.com/BoomerPsychosocialNeeds

December 21, 2011 by Eleanor Feldman Barbera, PhD

We've heard the rumblings of the coming generation in the voices of our "young" residents in their 50s and 60s. It's the younger residents who most often chafe at the restrictions of nursing home life, such as being unable to leave the facility unsupervised, or being cautioned to sit when they'd prefer to walk and take the risk of falling. As the baby boomers enter long-term care in greater numbers, those rumblings will grow louder, necessitating changes in how we deliver care. We'll be more successful in making these changes if we anticipate the needs of the boomers, rather than merely reacting to their dissatisfaction.

Attending to their psychosocial needs will help your boomers find comfort, enjoyment and purpose in their later years, thereby creating vital, thriving organizations better able to adapt to changes in the long-term care landscape. Here's what to look out for, and what you can do to help your organization and your clients:

1. Social connectedness

Internet access keeps boomer residents in touch with their social networks as well as the rest of the world. The next generation of residents will expect to be wired, so make your long-term care facility a hotspot now. To increase the value of this service, add adaptive equipment along with training in how to use it, lockable laptop drawers, additional electrical outlets, and policies on maintaining privacy in the nursing home.

2. Social differentiation

Say good-bye to "Goodnight, Irene" and hello to "You Can't Always Get What You Want", "Are You Lonesome Tonight?" and "Soldier Boy". The universal music of earlier generations shifted toward more individualized preferences in our new cohort, so plan on mixing your Motown with your Hendrix nights. Our boomers also had exposure to a wide variety of ethnic foods during their lifetimes. Consider polling residents to discover their preferences and offering an international option on your menu for greater variety and the opportunity for personal growth.

3. A platform for change

The activist generation doesn't believe that "the doctor knows best." This is a group of people used to fighting for their rights. Anticipate stronger resident councils looking to create concrete, positive change within your organization. Harnessing this power could be the best thing to ever happen to your community, because the residents will point to the changes you need to make to stay viable – the changes your line staff see but are afraid to tell you about. Give residents, and the staff members working with them, the tools to make it happen.

4. Consumer impulse

"'Consumerism Clashes with Measly Personal Needs Allowance' – story at 11." You can just envision the broadcast, right? It would go something like this:

"In today's news, a growing mob of elders in nursing homes across the country took to the Internet in protest of the PNA, which hasn't been increased since 1980. Here, a word from their leader, Ima Believer: 'We want an inflation adjustment! We want to have a place to buy things ourselves instead of having to rely on the kindness of strangers! We want debit cards linked to our accounts here at the home!'"

5. Continuing education

Opportunities for education can boost self-esteem and also create social connections. Boomers will be more likely to expect activities that provide possibilities for personal growth, such as classes on popular topics (like psychology) or activities that allow them to contribute to society. Take, for example, a bake sale to raise money for charity.

6. The boomer is always right

The service economy has made its mark on our upcoming group of residents. If a request for toileting is met with the often-overheard staff response, "Again?!" the boomer resident is far more likely to head over to the office of the Director of Nursing than to respond with the shamed silence or quiet seething of our current cohort of residents. Train your staff now on customer service techniques. Walk the floors on a regular basis listening to their interactions, and then train your staff again. Model appropriate behavior by speaking to staff members in the manner in which you want them to talk to residents.

7. Sex

Establish policies around sexual interactions and have your psychiatrists ready to evaluate for capacity to consent. Be prepared to discuss new relationships with family members – and get your multi-purpose room ready, because baby boomers are more likely than our current group of residents to expect to exercise their sexual freedom. Rehab referrals for this activity of daily living and requests for erectile dysfunction medication will become more common. Staff training will help your team handle residents' sexual concerns in a helpful and professional manner.

8. Fashion and décor

Floral back snap dresses with petal collars and sweatshirts with cute puppy prints will need to make way for more fashion-forward clothing designs that enhance the esteem of residents. And expect conservative room décor to be "tweaked" by younger residents. To make everyone happy, create a way for these adjustments to occur without destroying property, such as a system for easily changing artwork without putting holes in the walls. For example, consider adding molding close to the ceiling so that pictures can be hung with hooks or wires and no commitment. Or offer a variety of coordinated privacy curtains.

9. Scheduling daily priorities

Personal choice is important to boomer residents, making them more likely to demand flexible scheduling options than our current population. Imagine how empowered and cooperative residents would be if they had the opportunity to outline their schedules. "I'd like my wake-up call at 7:00 a.m., my breakfast between 7:30 and 8:00 a.m., and my rehab at 9:00 a.m." If we can work the nursing home schedule around the needs of the residents, rather than the residents around the needs of the nursing home, long-term care will become more livable.

10. Emotional support

Ageism among a group of residents that grew up with the rock and roll anthem lyric, "I hope I die before I get old," is likely to lead to challenges in self-concept for this generation. Support services, whether through individual psychotherapy or groups such as Alcoholics Anonymous or other illness-related organizations, will be expected by baby boomers, who are more aware of the mind-body connection and more comfortable sharing their concerns than our current residents.

Eleanor Feldman Barbera, PhD, is an author, speaker, and consultant on psychological issues in long-term care. For more information, visit Dr. Barbera's website, www.mybetternursinghome.com.

Section VI

When Should Activities Be Conducted with Clients?

Activities occur all day every day, and it is not so much a matter of when do you do them but about making every interaction memorable and focusing on a person as an individual. How you engage and what type of programs you do with Mr. Jones on Market Place Drive will not be the same for Mr. Smith of Main Street.

Centers for Medicare and Medicaid Service (CMS) define activities as follows: "Activities" refer to any endeavor, other than routine ADLs, in which a resident participates that is intended to enhance her/his sense of well-being and to promote or enhance physical, cognitive, and emotional health. These include, but are not limited to, activities that promote self-esteem, pleasure, comfort, education, creativity, success, and independence.

Based on the information one collects regarding a client's interests, a caregiver or family member can then begin to select activity programs that the client would enjoy. When choosing these programs, they must match the clients' physical, cognitive, and emotional abilities.

For many years, it was the philosophy of health care providers to make sure that activities are age appropriate. The thought process was that if someone is 80 years old, then the activities should be dignified and appropriate for what society perceives is appropriate for someone who is 80 years old. That thought process, as noble of a concept as it was, is certainly not practical. Let's look at that same 80-year-old client and factor in their cognitive status and diagnosis of dementia. Throughout the day, they are often asking for their mom and worrying about being late for school. One could conclude that if they are asking for their mom and worried about being late for school, that the person is cognitively fairly young and their activity program should consist of activities that one would do in school, such as math, reading, spelling, and possibly coloring. When creating an activity program, always ask, "Will this enhance their sense of well-being or promote or enhance physical, cognitive, and emotional health?"

While we are not suggesting treating a client like a child, we must understand their functional abilities and cognition, and then provide activity programs that would be reminiscent of what they did when they were in the prime of their life.

When choosing a program, do not be influenced by your perception of what an 80-year-old client should be doing. Your goal is to make each program person appropriate.

Person Appropriate

CMS states *person appropriate* refers to the idea that each resident has a personal identity and history that includes much more than just their medical illnesses or functional impairments, and that activities should be relevant – as much as possible – to the specific needs, interests, culture, background, etc., of the individual for whom they are developed.

Let's use gardening as an example of an activity. Person appropriate could mean different things to different people. Four people might all say they like gardening during their assessment, yet might not enjoy the same activity.

- Person 1 could enjoy going outside, cutting the grass, trimming the hedges, and weed whacking. Anything less would not meet their preference.
- Person 2 could enjoy planting flowers and vegetables and tending to their garden each day for an hour on their hands and knees.
- Person 3 could enjoy indoor plants – propagating plants and watering and caring for plants daily.
- Person 4 could enjoy arranging flowers in vases for table décor.

So one specific activity does not meet the individual interests of every client and therefore, when planning activities, ensure the activity is person appropriate. When a caregiver is conducting an assessment, the more details gathered from the client and/or their loved one, the more it will help in providing the needed information to develop an activity plan.

Activity programs should match the skills, abilities and preferences of the client with the demands of the activity and the characteristics of the physical, social, and cultural environments. Activities should encourage and enhance success and positive leisure experiences, regardless of functional level.

Before developing a person-centered activity plan, first discover who the person is as an individual. Develop questions to either ask or evaluate for the purpose of gathering appropriate information. Refer to the Personal History Form and Interest Page in Section VIII. This evaluation becomes the Life History Assessment.

- Previous occupations
    - When gathering information, get specific names of companies they worked for throughout their employment history along with any further details such as

where companies were located, what type of work they did, and names of coworkers or supervisors. All of these details can become talking points with caregivers and family members. If the client has cognitive loss, then it becomes even more important to know the details of the occupation. When a caregiver knows this information and is able to articulate the details to a client, it creates a bonding experience and fosters a relationship of both trust and security.

- Places traveled
    - If the client and or their family have pictures of their traveling experiences, have the family members write all of the identifying information on the backs of the pictures. What year were the pictures taken? Where was the picture taken? Have the family member write the names and relationships of the people in the picture. Pictures with stories are a wonderful way of creating a past experience with a client. Without the identifying information, the caregiver has to ask the client for those details, and often the client does not remember.

- Hobbies
    - During the assessment process, it is helpful to find out hobbies that not only the client participates in or enjoys now, but also enjoyed throughout his/her lifetime.
    - Remember when choosing activity programs, the client most likely has a stronger long-term memory and will enjoy focusing on hobbies they did when their memories are the strongest.

- Adaptations/modifications needed
    - Any activity can be modified or adapted to a level where the client can succeed.
    - Never say, "Oh, she can't do that anymore." Instead say, "OK. She likes this activity and she has these abilities." or "How can I modify this so she can enjoy it?"
    - Use the client's available abilities.

- Ability to make their needs known
    - Needs can be made known either verbally or nonverbally.
    - Observation is a key tool when working with a client who can no longer make their needs known.
    - Nurses use the terminology "will anticipate needs," which describes what caregivers will do for their client.

- Observe the client's reaction to tasks by observing their facial expressions, breathing patterns, and behaviors. This observation will provide insight into contentment, boredom, or frustration.

– Talents/passions
    - The assessment process is the key to successful programming.
    - Help the family understand to tell their loved one's story; no detail is too small.
    - Knowing a client's passions as a healthier individual will provide the key to unlock memories and aid in recreating past life experiences.

– Client strengths
    - Move away from the medical model of care, which focuses on sick, old, frail or having a deficit. Instead, move into a social model using Florence Nightingale's theory, which suggests treating the medical condition as well as the soul.
    - List the client's strengths and empower the client to utilize their strengths on a daily basis.
    - By empowering a person, you increase their confidence, self-esteem, and overall psychosocial well-being.

– Typical day now
    - Discover what comprises a typical day for the client. It is an important question to ask, so if your intent is to make changes to increase a client's stimulation and productivity, do so in a gradual and goal-directed way, giving the control to the client with your power of persuasion. In other words, give the client a reason to get out of bed or get dressed to complete a task. As human beings, we have the need to feel useful and purposeful, so if you can provide a client with that reason, utilizing knowledge, values, and past experiences, your client's quality of life will increase and your families will be satisfied.

– Typical day then
    - It is important to recreate the client's former experiences daily. If the client is a person who gets up early, makes a light breakfast, completes light chores, and tends to the garden then, if medically appropriate, all attempts should be made to keep the client as active as possible to the fullest extent.

- Family tree –
    - Support a client to share his/her family genealogy. Using technology like the Internet and websites, such as www.ancestry.com, is a great way to share information that the client has and also expand the information as he/she learns new and exciting information about his/her past.
    - It is just as important to know the relationships that are important to the client – both human and animal. As discussed in the last section, engaging a client and needing to know intimate details becomes more relevant if you have a client who believes he/she is a young teenager and is looking for "Max." You might think Max is a friend and respond "Max is in church," but if Max is the client's childhood dog, then you aren't able to give an answer that makes sense to the client. As a result, you begin to foster distrust which could cause behavioral issues.

- Present behaviors – Use A-B-C behavior management. (Refer to Section II.)
    - Having a caregiver or health care professional who knows the information on potential behavior issues, trigger, and intervention could prevent an occurrence.
    - A caregiver may observe that Mrs. Smith is typically pleasant and easygoing. But when the soap operas are on TV, she becomes agitated and visibly anxious as evidenced by wringing her hands and being tearful. Clients who are cognitively impaired could begin to have a problem distinguishing between what is real and what is not real on TV. Mrs. Smith might believe that these are real people dealing with such tragedy and drama that she, herself, begins to share those feelings. Now as a caregiver, you are aware of this key piece of information and can ensure that Mrs. Smith is not around the TV when these types of programs are being viewed.
    - Behaviors, triggers, and interventions should be information that travels with the client throughout his/her health care journey. Each health care setting has its unique strengths, and with those strengths also come weaknesses.

***In an acute hospital setting, the focus is on treating the medical need that resulted in the hospitalization. They do not focus on client emotional needs so, if the hospital did not have this behavioral information, an unsuspecting aide could turn on the TV to the soaps while the client is being treated for agitation or aggression. This treatment typically comes in the form of antipsychotic drugs or, in worst-case scenario, restraints.

Family members and home care caregivers are the ones who know the client in the most comfortable setting and have knowledge of every aspect of the client. Never think that the piece of information you have is not relevant or not important.

- Client spiritual/inspirational interests needed:
  - Knowing the client's religious affiliation is important, but in these areas we are also addressing spirituality and inspiration.
  - Religious affiliation should include not only the affiliation but also the name of the church, synagogue, etc., they attended (if applicable), as well as names of key religious members. Certain affiliations use specific scriptures at pivotal life events, including music played during a service. For example, one affiliation may sing "Amazing Grace" as a source of happiness and inspiration, while another affiliation may only play that song at funerals. If your intent is to play religious music to inspire, then you will need to know what songs in that religion meet that need.
  - If you meet a client who has a religious affiliation that you do not have knowledge of, take the opportunity to have the client explain their belief system. You also can use the Internet to conduct research. Just remember, by helping a client participate in a religious act that may be different from your belief system, it does not take away from your own personal belief.
  - Spirituality has nothing to do with religion, but often people think it is interchangeable.
    - According to *Psychology Today,* the term "spirituality" lacks a conclusive definition, although social scientists have defined spirituality as the search for "the sacred," where "the sacred" is broadly defined as "that which is set apart from the ordinary and worthy of veneration."
    - The use of the term "spirituality" has changed throughout the years. Today, spirituality is often separated from religion, and contains a blend of humanistic psychology with traditions aimed at personal well-being and personal development. In Section I, we talked about Maslow's Hierarchy of Needs and human psychological development. In relation, it can be viewed that a person's spiritual development mirrors the higher aspects of the pyramid of development.

- Client's hopes and dreams
    - Taken right from the movie *The Bucket List,* people often have a list of hopes and dreams of things they would like to do before they pass on to the next life.
    - Ask a client to identify some of the things they want to do before it is their time or while they still have time. You might be surprised at the answers. It can be as simple as writing a letter to the president of the United States or riding a camel.
    - There is a nonprofit company called Second Wind Dreams whose mission is to change the perception of aging one dream at a time. It is much more than a nonprofit organization. Second Wind Dreams considers itself a movement to bring seniors back to the forefront of our society and make them feel special.

    For more information about getting involved in Second Wind Dreams or making a client's dream come true contact:
    - Second Wind Dreams
      4343 Shallowford Road, Suite E6
      Marietta, GA 30062
      1-678-624-0500
      www.secondwind.org

Case Study

Case Study of successful interaction and engagement of activities

Mr. Bob has Alzheimer's and lives with his wife. His wife has a caregiver that comes in everyday to help keep him stimulated and engaged. The frustration is that he has limited cognition and short-term memory loss. During the standardized assessment, the intake nurse asked the spouse, "How does Bob spend his day?" Mary responded, "He sleeps … he does not have any hobbies … he can't do anything, he doesn't remember anything..." The caregiver had no real information provided to assist her in the development of a daily activity program for Bob. Through a series of "yes" and "no" questions, the caregiver was still unable to obtain any true information.

One day, Bob's daughter, who lived out of town and worked in the health care industry, came to visit and was frustrated with the caregiver because her father was no more engaged with a caregiver than he was with his wife. During the conversation, the caregiver reviewed the information she had obtained about Bob and the daughter began to tell Bob's story. The daughter stated that her dad was an army man who nearly went to Vietnam, but the week before deployment the war ended. She shared with the caregiver that her dad still has several military boxes in the shed that contain everything from his uniform to medals to other important trinkets and treasures. She explained that frequently in her life, she remembers her dad pulling out those boxes and telling her hours upon hours of stories related to the time he spent in boot camp in North Carolina.

The daughter began to write a list of discussion topics related to his army days that would elicit conversation with her dad. The daughter then decided that she would get her brothers and sisters to write their fondest memories and stories about Bob. She planned to put them in a binder so the caregiver would have something to talk about, in hopes that this would engage Bob in conversation and motivate him to be more active. By the end of her visit, she provided the caregiver with a binder that contained stories and pictures and also assembled "memory boxes" that coincided with those stories.

Within the next week, Bob was engaged and talking and active every day. The caregiver began to write the interactions and new details revealed by Bob so the book would also serve as Bob's legacy and would be shared with Bob's grandchildren when they visited. Even Bob's wife, Mary, felt a renewed connection with her husband because he was talking to her again and they would talk and laugh for hours. As a result, the caregiver was not frustrated and enjoyed coming to work everyday to learn more about Bob. Mary began to tell her husband's story and the library of information grew daily.

Person-Directed Care and Continuity of Care

The American Medical Director Association defines person-directed care as "a philosophy that encourages both older adults and their caregivers to express choice and proactive self-determination in meaningful ways at every level of daily life. Values are essential to this philosophy, which involves choice, dignity, respect, self-determination, and personal living."

The home health industry again is at an advantage to other health care industries because they are seeing clients in the early stage of requiring assistance. This may be the starting point for caregivers to assist the client in voicing their preferences and choices as well as developing a plan that can follow them throughout the continuum of care.

Continuity of care is the key element of success to person-directed care. Through communication and management, a client's wishes and directions are followed with them through all aspect of the health care system. A person-customary routine and personal preference typically remains unchanged with the expectation to the level of assistance one needs to maintain these preferences.

Successful continuity of care is achieved regardless of changes in health status, health care service providers, or settings. Families and clients judge continuity of care by their perception that health care staff has sufficient knowledge and information about them as an individual (as obtained from prior health care providers) and continues to develop a plan that meets both client and family goals while maintaining their individualized version of quality of life.

Continuity of care, as it relates to the activity arena, maintains a person's individuality. Regardless of the health care provider or setting in which services are rendered, that person's preferences and customary routines are factored in when developing a plan of care.

The health care industry is now responding to the demand set by clients and their families, and has made their focus on person-directed health which will achieve a balanced set of outcomes related to improved client/family services, provider experience, and improved quality of life. In the long term, the assessment and regulatory survey process has begun to move from a staff perspective of care to a client perspective model, thus giving the client a voice in how care is provided and what degree of satisfaction it provides to the client.

Successful Integrated Care

Integrated care is also known as coordinated care or comprehensive care. It is becoming a national trend in health care reforms and is now becoming the organization focus of many companies. Integrated care may be seen as a response to the fragmented delivery of health and social services that has been a major complaint with the health care system.

Even though there are many definitions of integrated health care, integration is a means to improve services in relation to access, quality, user satisfaction, and efficiency.

Integrated care distinguishes different ways and degrees of working together. The concept of *continuity of care* is closely related to integrated care; it emphasizes the patient's perspective through the system of health and social services, providing valuable lessons for the integration of systems. The concept of integrated care seems particularly important to service provisions to the elderly, as elderly patients often are chronically ill and subject to co-morbidities, and thus in special need of continuous care.

The two most well-known examples of integrated health care are the United States Department of Veterans Affairs (largest integrated care delivery system in the U.S.) and managed health care company Kaiser Permanente (largest private U.S. health care system).

Customary Routines and Preferences

Centers for Medicare and Medicaid Services (CMS) has developed uniform guidelines for completing the Minimum Data Set (MDS). The MDS is completed for skilled nursing facilities as a comprehensive assessment. Many years of research conclude that giving the client a voice in directing their preference and care results in better quality of care and preservation of the individuality of a person. Despite where a client is receiving supportive services, the philosophy of giving the client a voice (planning their days and goals around information obtained to create an individualized plan based on the client's preferences) has proven successful. This evaluation process gives your client a voice in his/her care.

As the health care arena strives to develop consistency with care and the flow of information, it is beneficial to integrate the language used in long-term care facilities within our communication through the continuity of care.

The MDS evaluates client preferences in several areas. For the purpose of developing a daily plan of care, we will be discussing two areas: daily customary routine and activity preferences. The goal is to gain from the client's perspective how important certain aspects of care and activity interests are to them as an individual.

Daily Customary Routine

Item Rationale – Why it's important to know

- Clients have a distinct lifestyle preference and it should be preserved to the greatest extent possible. All reasonable accommodations should be made to maintain lifestyle preferences.
- A lack of lifestyle preferences can contribute to a depressed mood and increased behavior symptoms. When a person feels like their control has been removed and his/her preferences are not respected as an individual, it can be demoralizing.

Areas to Gain Client's Preference

- Choosing clothing
    - Knowing a client's preference and encouraging them to participate in the process of selecting clothing can be empowering to a client.
    - A caregiver must become familiar with a client's clothing preference. Do they enjoy lounging in sweatpants and slippers or are they meticulous about having matching outfits and coordinating down to the accessories they choose?
    - Do they have a favorite article of clothing or accessory that they must wear?

- Choosing bed time
    - Discover the client's evening routine. Is it a hot shower, warm cup of milk, and watching the evening news before settling in? Or is it a regimented 9:00 p.m. bed time?
    - Gaining this information can help alleviate stress, which could result in a client not sleeping or a client falling because they were put to bed too early or their nightly routine was not followed.

- Eating snacks between meals
    - Find out how important it is to a client to have snacks between meals – specifically the client's preference. Diabetics are a separate issue. Does the client enjoy something sweet in the evening? Or is the client very health conscious and enjoy fresh vegetables and cheese after lunch and before dinner?
    - The focus is assisting the client in maintaining the same routine as when they were completely independent.

- Interest level with involving family in care discussions
    - As long as your client is competent, alert, and oriented, they should be given the right to dictate who receives information about their health care status.
    - Knowing the client's preference and then respecting that preference will foster a trusting and caring relationship.

Activity Preferences

As part of the assessment, the Personal History Form and Interest Page become the basis for the client's activities and leisure interests. When the form is completed accurately, it will detail if an activity is a leisure pursuit that the client engaged in previously, if it is something they are currently doing, or if it is something they expressed an interest in learning. No matter when the interest developed, it gives you the recipe for what to do now.

Item Rationale: Why do I need to know what they enjoy?

- Activities are a way for individuals to establish meaning in their lives, and the need for enjoyable activities does not change based on age or health needs. The only thing that changes is the level of assistance they may need to engage in those pursuits.

- A lack of opportunity to engage in meaningful and enjoyable activities can result in boredom, depression, and behavioral disturbances. This is what our families complain about to the staff. They can no longer get their loved one to engage in life activities. This disengagement causes depression and frustration between the caregiver and the client, which then could result in behavioral disturbances. We are human, and it is in our nature to be productive to the extent we desire.

- Individuals vary in the activities they prefer, reflecting unique personalities, past interests, perceived environmental constraints, religious and cultural background, and changing physical and mental abilities. Health care providers have a great opportunity to empower a client to see that they possess many great talents and abilities, and to modify or adapt the activity to allow engagement at an independent level, essentially restoring their self-esteem and self-worth.

Activity Programming Related to Medical Care Areas

Activity engagement encompasses much more than keeping someone occupied throughout the day. Activities are an important therapeutic modality in the health care provided. An ongoing, meaningful activity program can help address, redirect, or eliminate many medical conditions.

During the initial assessment or intake evaluation, many care areas are medically evaluated to determine such areas as visual abilities, hearing abilities, and physical and mental abilities. All of these care areas have a significant relationship to activity programming. Below you will find a list of care areas that one might find in a client and how activity interventions could be beneficial.

Delirium – This acute, confused state is a syndrome that presents as severe confusion and disorientation, developing with a relatively rapid onset and fluctuating in intensity. It is a syndrome which occurs more frequently in people in their later years. Much research has been conducted that states meaningful, individualized activity programs help prevent further decline and improve quality of life while the problem is being treated.

Cognitive Loss/Dementia – Activities that provide positive experiences and are modified to individual abilities help the client participate at their highest practicable level. A caregiver should introduce activities that are based on a comprehensive evaluation and enhance a client's quality of life. If a client has a cognitive impairment, modify the activity and/or break down instructions to a task that is easier to accomplish.

Communication Barriers – Use nonverbal communication along with the spoken word. For more information, please refer to Section II. Identify the client's barriers, and then devise a plan that addresses these barriers, resulting in good communication techniques for the client.

Psychosocial Well-Being – With every client interaction, we must ask. "How does this affect their psychosocial well-being?" This includes the words you choose in a response to the types of interactions and activities provided. Caregivers provide social relationships while conducting activities to address cognitive/communication deficits. When treating a client like an individual and focusing on the psychosocial well-being, the root cause of the lack of interest in engaging socially with others becomes clear.

Depressed Mood – Depression and psychosocial well-being go hand in hand. There are many factors that can contribute to this issue. Consistent approaches, utilizing the life review to individualize activity programs, and modifying and adapting each activity to promote independence means that a client is less likely to become depressed. Encourage your client to tell their story.

Behaviors – Keep in mind that behaviors are nothing more than a means to communicate what the client can no longer say with words. Caregivers are charged with balancing the stimulation a client receives to helping manage anxiety, fear, boredom, or frustration, which can all manifest as a challenging behavior. When faced with a difficult behavior, develop a behavior management plan that can be utilized consistently with both family and caregivers. Introduce activities that will teach those coping skills as well as relaxation and anger management techniques. Keep activities short in duration and repetitious.

Evaluation/Reassessment Activity Analysis

Activity analysis is defined by Crepau (1996) as "the process by which an activity is broken down into its component parts to determine the skills required to do it."

Ensuring that the activity matches a client's ability or interest is just as important as ensuring the medication dose given to a client matches the prescribed amount. If an activity is too difficult, the client may be frustrated, give up, and withdraw – more as a result of being faced with yet another task that the person cannot accomplish. If the activity does not stimulate the client, he/she may not even attempt to participate in the activity program.

Completing an activity analysis can determine if the activity is appropriate for the client's ability. During this analysis, the facilitator can make changes to the activity lesson plan by adding in variation, suggesting adaptive equipment, or suggesting verbal cueing that was successful with the client during the activity lesson. We use this tool to assist in the selection of appropriate activities and modifications.

The activity analysis begins with the written lesson plan – listing the steps necessary for facilitating this activity with your client. The lesson plan may start as a generic template. After a program is conducted, it is important for the facilitator to write suggestions to the next facilitator in the evaluation area of the lesson plan. For example, "Client needs verbal cueing throughout the program." The evaluation is now what turns this generic activity into a person-specific activity program.

While determining when to schedule activities, establish a baseline understanding for person-directed care, continuity of care, and customary routine and preferences. From that core knowledge come the tools to develop an individualized plan for each client.

Summary

Every endeavor outside the pursuits of daily living is considered an activity. Your client will be successful and happy once you identify their life history, customary routines, and individual preferences.

Engaging a client in meaningful, individualized activities can combat loneliness, boredom, and depression. Use the tools provided in this manual to be better prepared to understand and manage each client. When confronted with an issue, take a step back and review the information provided about the client. Then try something new. Not every attempt will be successful, but remember, you are holding a whole arsenal of information at your fingertips.

This process of customizing activities for each client will continue to be ongoing and ever-changing. Caring for a human being is, at times, most challenging. But at the same time, it can be the most rewarding experience. You are entrusted with a gift. That gift is assisting a person live their life one day at a time.

Section VII

Sample Activities

This section provides sample activities in a Lesson Plan format to use with clients. As with any plan, this is meant as a guideline, and each of your clients' abilities and responses will dictate how to modify/adapt each lesson plan to meet their individual needs and abilities. The lesson plan should be an ever-changing plan. It is meant to be written on to note the changes made from the original plan so the next person working with the client can follow your modifications with the intent of recreating positive experiences.

Use the blank Lesson Plan template to develop client-specific activities by completing the log and developing an individualized activity library.

How to Use Lesson Plan

Date	Document the date activity is used with the client
Program Name	Activity name or client-preferred activity name
Objective of Activity	To provide meaningful, purposeful activities that will engage clients
Materials	Suggested materials/resources to use with this program
Prerequisite Skills	Physical skills/abilities a client should possess to engage in a particular program
Activity Outline	Step-by-step instructions to complete the program
Evaluation	A thorough evaluation is the most important part of the lesson plan. When doing an activity with the client, record any verbal cues, assistance, or modifications to incorporate. It is also helpful to include the client's response to the program. Note if the client dislikes a certain activity and won't ever be interested in engaging in this activity in the future. Note programs that are successful at distracting or eliminating a negative behavior (diversional activities). Encourage family members and caregivers to use the evaluation section and also to leave tips. Don't waste time recreating the wheel of knowledge; pass on the information so everyone presents the program in the same way with the same modifications and cueing, and achieving the same positive outcomes.

Lesson Plan

Date:	Program Name:

Objective of Activity
- ➢
- ➢
- ➢
- ➢
- ➢

Materials
- ➢
- ➢
- ➢
- ➢
- ➢
- ➢

Prerequisite Skills
- ➢
- ➢
- ➢
- ➢

Activity Outline

Evaluation

Lesson Plan

Date:	**Program Name:** Trivia / Crossword Puzzles / Code Breakers / Word Scramble

Objective of Activity
- Stimulate cognitive functioning
- Increase self-worth
- Increase socialization through shared experiences
- Stimulate memory
- Provide an opportunity for reminiscing

Materials
- R.O.S. *BIG Book*
- R.O.S. *How Much Do You Know About* Series (match the topic with clients' interests)
-
-
-
-

Prerequisite Skills
- Listening skills
- Motor skills
-
-

Activity Outline

You can use this activity as an independent project or work on it together with the client. This activity can be conducted either verbally or written.

1. Explain to clients that they should complete the phrase or answer the question, depending on the type of trivia.
2. Encourage clients to change stories related to the topics you are discussing.
3. Allow ample time for clients to process the question.
4. You may have to repeat the question a second time in the exact way you asked it the first time.
5. Ask each question two times before giving them the answer.
6. Give much praise for each answer, regardless if they are correct.

Evaluation

Lesson Plan

Date:	**Program Name:** Name That Object

Objective of Activity
- Stimulate cognitive functioning
- Increase socialization through shared experiences
- Promote verbal skills
- Provide a sense of accomplishment in performance

Materials
- None

Prerequisite Skills
- Listening skills

Activity Outline

Ask participants to name the object to the best of their ability. (If your client can't immediately answer, begin giving clues until he/she guesses the answer.)

1. A piece of clothing that keeps your hands warm
2. Something to drink that has Vitamin C
3. An animal that has a bad odor
4. A vehicle that transports people in an emergency
5. A place where planes take off and land
6. The color of the grass and leaves
7. A part of the body that bends
8. Something used to see in the dark
9. A material used to build houses
10. Something used to write on a blackboard
11. A room that has a sink, stove, and refrigerator
12. A place to buy fuel for a car
13. A shape with four corners
14. Something used to get wrinkles out of clothes
15. A holiday where we can see fireworks
16. A place to buy watches, earrings, and rings
17. Something that tells the month and year
18. A dessert that can have frosting
19. Something to put on a cut
20. Something that transports a wrecked car

Evaluation

Lesson Plan

Date:	**Program Name:** Opposites Attract

Objective of Activity
- Stimulate cognitive functioning
- Increase socialization through shared experiences
- Promote verbal skills
- Provide a sense of accomplishment in performance

Materials
- None

Prerequisite Skills
- Listening skills

Activity Outline

Have participants finish these well-known opposites. Answers are in parenthesis.

1. Up____ (down)
2. Out ____ (in)
3. Dark _____ (light)
4. Soft_____ (hard)
5. Front_____ (back)
6. Black _____ (white)
7. Inhale_____ (exhale)
8. Rise_____ (fall)
9. Good_____ (bad)
10. Fast_____ (slow)
11. Before_____ (after)
12. East_____ (west)
13. Stop_____ (go)
14. Cold_____ (hot)
15. Night_____ (day)
16. Happy_____ (sad)
17. Big _____ (small)
18. Sunny _____ (rainy), (cloudy)
19. Wrong_____ (right)
20. Tall_____ (short)

Evaluation

Lesson Plan

Date:	**Program Name:** Animal Trivia

Objective of Activity
- Stimulate cognitive functioning
- Stimulate spiritual, intellectual, and emotional discussion
- Promote visual and verbal skills
- Provide a sense of accomplishment in performance
- Provide an opportunity for reminiscing

Materials
- None

Prerequisite Skills
- Listening skills

Activity Outline

Have participants guess the well-known animals.

1. Builds a dam… (Beaver)
2. Swings from trees… (Monkey)
3. Gallops and bucks… (Horse)
4. Has orange stripes… (Tiger)
5. The biggest land animal… (Elephant)
6. Barks and do tricks… (Dog)
7. Hops around Australia… (Kangaroo)
8. Hides nuts for winter…(Squirrel)
9. Beats on its chest… (Gorilla)
10. Eats the highest leaves from the tree… (Giraffe)
11. Has a hump… (Camel)
12. Carries its house on its back… (Turtle)
13. Flies at night and sleeps upside down during the day…(Bat)
14. Spins cobwebs… (Spider)
15. Has a large white stripe down the center of its back…(Skunk)
16. Has black and white stripes…(Zebra)
17. Slithers up trees and on the ground…(Snake)
18. The first animal in space…(Chimpanzee)
19. Known for laughing…(Hyena)
20. Flies with Santa… (Reindeer)

Evaluation

Lesson Plan

Date:	**Program Name:** Awareness Ribbon Color

Objective of Activity
- Maintain/increase fine motor stimulation
- Opportunity for reflection and relaxation
- Promote fine motor skills
- Stimulate memory
- Provide an opportunity for reminiscing

Materials
- Ribbon template
- Crayons, colored pencils or markers

Prerequisite Skills
- Motor skills
- Hand movement
- Hand-eye coordination

Activity Outline

For awareness, have participants engage in this coloring activity.

Use the ribbon template provided and the awareness chart.

Have participants choose their cause and color the ribbon with the coordinating color.

Evaluation

Awareness Ribbon Color Guide

Ribbon Color	Awareness / Cause
Black	Skin Cancer
	Sleep Apnea
Blue	Arthritis
	Colon Cancer
	Crohn's Disease
	Huntington's Disease
	Rectal Cancer
	Reye's Syndrome
Blue and Yellow	Down Syndrome
Burgundy	Brain Aneurysm
	Disabled Adults
	Hospice Care
Burgundy and Ivory	Oral Cancer
	Head Cancer
	Neck Cancer
Gold	Childhood Cancer (alternate colors: pink & light blue)
	COPD
	Pediatric Cancer
Gray	Brain Cancer
	Brain Tumors
	Diabetes
	Mental Illness
Green	Bipolar Disorder
	Cerebral Palsy
	Depression
	Kidney Disease
	Leukemia
	Organ Donation
Lime Green	Lymphoma
	Muscular Dystrophy
Orange	Hunger
	Leukemia
	Lupus
	Multiple Sclerosis (MS)
Pink	Breast Cancer
Pinstripe	Lou Gehrig's Disease
Purple	Alzheimer's Disease
Puzzle	Autism
Red	AIDS and HIV
	Congenital Heart Disease
	Congestive Heart Failure
Red, White and Blue	Patriotism
	9/11 Heroes
Yellow	General Symbol for Hope
	POW/MIA (alternate color: black)

Lesson Plan

Date:	**Program Name:** Crossword

Objective of Activity
- Maintain/increase sequencing skills
- Stimulate cognitive functioning
- Increase socialization through shared experiences
- Promote fine motor skills
- Provide a sense of accomplishment in performance

Materials
- R.O.S. *BIG Book*

Prerequisite Skills
- Listening skills
- Hand-eye coordination

Activity Outline

Have participants answer questions to the best of their ability.

In this fun and easy crossword, have participants think of the Halloween-themed answers.

Evaluation

Lesson Plan

Date:	**Program Name:** Juice Box Mummy

Objective of Activity

- Maintain/increase sequencing skills
- Stimulate cognitive functioning
- Maintain/increase fine motor stimulation
- Promote fine motor skills
- Provide a sense of accomplishment in performance

Materials

- Empty juice box container
- 2 tablespoons rice
- Sandwich bag
- Tape
- Black and white construction paper
- Scissors
- Glue stick
- 2 medium googly eyes
- White craft glue

Prerequisite Skills

- Listening skills
- Motor skills
- Hand movement
- Hand-eye coordination

Activity Outline

Have participants get in the Halloween spirit by making this festive craft.

1. Open the top of the juice box container. Rinse and dry thoroughly.
2. Place rice inside sandwich bag. Roll up the bag and secure with tape. (Or use a sandwich bag with a zip enclosure.) Place the bag of rice inside the juice box and tape the top closed.
3. Cut a piece of black construction paper, large enough to cover the top half of the front of the juice box. Glue it in place.
4. Tear white construction paper in strips and glue them around the box, leaving a small section of the black paper visible.
5. Use white craft glue to attach two googly eyes to the black paper.

Evaluation

Lesson Plan

Date:	**Program Name:** Pom-pom Spiders

Objective of Activity
- Maintain/increase sequencing skills
- Stimulate cognitive functioning
- Maintain/increase fine motor stimulation
- Promote fine motor skills
- Provide a sense of accomplishment in performance
- Provide an opportunity for reminiscing

Materials
- Yarn
- Scissors
- 4 chenille stems
- Scrap cardboard
- Googly eyes
- Glue
- Pom-poms

Prerequisite Skills
- Listening skills
- Motor skills
- Hand movement
- Hand-eye coordination

Activity Outline

Have participants get into the Halloween spirit by making festive spiders.

1. Cut a piece of yarn about 2 feet long. (Set aside.)
2. Cut a piece of scrap cardboard about 3 inches long by 2 inches wide.
3. Wrap about a yard or two of yarn lengthwise around the rectangular piece of cardboard. (Wrap yarn slightly loose for easy removal from the cardboard.)
4. Carefully slide the yarn from the cardboard, keeping the yarn loops in place.
5. Place 4 chenille stems over the loops. Tightly tie the 2-foot piece of yarn around the middle of the loops and chenille stems.
6. Cut the yarn loops at their edges. Trim the pom-pom so that it makes a nice circle, and then glue it to the yarn loops.
7. Bend the spider's legs and glue on the googly eyes.

Evaluation

Lesson Plan

Date:	**Program Name:** Talent Show

Objective of Activity
- Increase socialization through shared experiences
- Opportunity for reflection and relaxation
- Stimulate past experience
- Increased socialization
- Foster friendship, laughter, and closeness
- Provide a sense of accomplishment in performance
- Raise self-esteem

Materials
- Sheet music
- Piano
- Music

Prerequisite Skills
- Listening skills
- Motor skills

Activity Outline

For piano month, have participants engage in a talent show.

Have participants bring their favorite songs Have participants engage in a sing-a-long.

Participants can also show off any other talents.

Evaluation

Lesson Plan

Date:	**Program Name:** Bird Watching

Objective of Activity
- Promote/enhance sensory awareness
- Stimulate spiritual, intellectual, and emotional discussion
- Visual, auditory, and tactile stimulation
- Opportunity for reflection and relaxation
- Provide an opportunity for reminiscing

Materials
- Look on the internet for pictures of various birds that live in your geographical area.

Prerequisite Skills
- Listening skills
- Motor skills
- Hand movement
- Hand-eye coordination

Activity Outline

Have participants identify different birds in the area while on their walks.

Take the participants on long or short walks around the facility, to the courtyard or around their neighborhood and have them watch birds.

Evaluation

Lesson Plan

Date:	**Program Name:** Cherry Kool-Aid Paint

Objective of Activity
- Maintain/increase sequencing skills
- Stimulate cognitive functioning
- Maintain/increase fine motor stimulation
- Promote fine motor skills
- Provide a sense of accomplishment in performance

Materials
- 2 packages unsweetened cherry Kool-Aid
- 2 cups flour
- ½ cup salt
- 3 cups boiling water
- 3 tablespoons oil
- Card stock paper
- Paintbrushes

Prerequisite Skills
- Listening skills
- Motor skills
- Hand movement
- Hand-eye coordination

Activity Outline

For Cherry Month, have participants make some fun paint to decorate pictures.

1. Mix unsweetened mix, flour, and salt. Then add boiling water and oil.
2. Use this fun paint on card stock paper or construction paper.

Evaluation

Lesson Plan

Date:	**Program Name:** Spring Planting

Objective of Activity

- Promote/enhance sensory awareness
- Maintain/increase sequencing skills
- Maintain/increase fine motor stimulation
- Visual, auditory and tactile stimulation
- Opportunity for reflection and relaxation
- Stimulate past experience
- Provide an opportunity for reminiscing

Materials

- Flower seeds
- Soil
- Flower pots
- Water
- Small shovels or large spoons
- R.O.S. Therapy Systems Legacy Kit with insert for planting

Prerequisite Skills

- Listening skills
- Motor skills
- Hand movement
- Hand-eye coordination

Activity Outline

For the start of spring, have participants plant flowers in their own flower pots.

1. Help participants put soil into their flower pots.
2. Dig a hole(s) to plant seeds.
3. Put seeds in the hole(s) and cover with soil.
4. Water the plant as needed so participants can watch their flowers grow.

Evaluation

Lesson Plan

Date:	**Program Name:** Frozen Yogurt Party

Objective of Activity
- Increase self-worth
- Increase socialization through shared experiences
- Stimulate spiritual, intellectual, and emotional discussion
- Opportunity for reflection and relaxation
- Increased socialization
- Increase appetite
- Raise self-esteem

Materials
- Frozen yogurt
- Yogurt toppings
- Bowls
- Spoons
- Napkins

Prerequisite Skills
- Listening skills
- Hand eye coordination

Activity Outline

Have participants get involved in a frozen yogurt party.

Serve participants their favorite flavors and toppings. Add some music to the festivities and display artwork created this month.

Evaluation

Lesson Plan

Date:	**Program Name:** Tissue Paper Butterflies

Objective of Activity

- Maintain/increase sequencing skills
- Stimulate cognitive functioning
- Maintain/increase fine motor stimulation
- Promote fine motor skills
- Provide a sense of accomplishment in performance
- Stimulate memory
- Provide an opportunity for reminiscing

Materials

- 2 - 4 inch x 4 inch pieces of tissue paper
- Scissors
- Chenille stem
- String or thread

Prerequisite Skills

- Listening skills
- Motor skills
- Hand movement
- Hand-eye coordination

Activity Outline

Have participants create tissue paper butterflies.

1. Stack the 2 tissue squares.
2. Trim the edges so they look like wings.
3. Fold the chenille stem in half over the wings, bunching the tissue slightly.
4. Twist together the chenille stem ends to hold the paper in place. Then curl the chenille stem tips around your finger to create antennae.
5. Tie one end of the thread or string to the chenille stem to hang the butterfly.

Evaluation

Lesson Plan

Date:	Program Name: Dominoes

Objective of Activity

- Maintain/increase sequencing skills
- Stimulate cognitive functioning
- Stimulate past experience
- Promote visual and verbal skills
- Provide a sense of accomplishment in performance
- Raise self-esteem

Materials

- Several packs of large-dot dominoes (at least 5 dominoes per participant)

Prerequisite Skills

- Listening skills
- Motor skills
- Hand movement
- Hand-eye coordination

Activity Outline

1. Introduce yourself to the group.
2. Explain to participants that you will distribute the dominoes evenly among the group.
3. Have participants create a chain of dominoes by matching the number on each end of the dominoes.
4. Give praise and encouragement throughout the activity.
5. If necessary, help participants find the correct dominoes.

Evaluation

Lesson Plan

Date:	Program Name: Baking/Cooking

Objective of Activity

- Promote/enhance sensory awareness
- Maintain/increase sequencing skills
- Increase socialization through shared experiences
- Visual, auditory, and tactile stimulation
- Stimulate past experience
- Sensory stimulation
- Increase appetite
- Foster friendship, laughter, and closeness
- Provide a sense of accomplishment in performance
- Raise self-esteem
- Stimulate memory
- Provide an opportunity for reminiscing

Materials

- Supplies depend upon recipe, ingredients, and necessary cooking utensils.
- Latex gloves

Prerequisite Skills

- Listening skills
- Motor Skills
- Hand movement
- Hand-eye coordination

Activity Outline

1. Have all participants wash hands.
2. Assist them with applying latex gloves.
3. Read the recipe to the group, and then assign participants to a specific task to make the recipe. (Always consider participants' abilities.)
4. Follow recipe directions.
5. Encourage discussion and reminiscing.
6. Serve refreshments with the food just prepared.
7. If the recipe requires a lengthy cooking time, have a prepared version ready to eat.

Evaluation

Section VIII

Resources

Resources for Products and Education

<u>*R.O.S. Therapy Systems*</u> – The mission of R.O.S. Therapy Systems is to Improve Quality of Life through Activities and Education.

www.ROSTherapySystems.com
Toll-Free: 888-352-9788
Email: info@ROSTherapySystems.com

<u>*Alzheimer's Association*</u> – The Alzheimer's Association works on global, national and local levels to enhance care for, and support all those affected by Alzheimer's and related dementias.

www.alz.org
Toll-Free: 800-272-3900
TDD: 866-403-3073
Email: info@alz.org

<u>*National Parkinson Foundation*</u> – The mission of the National Parkinson Foundation is simple – to improve the lives of people with Parkinson's disease through research, education and outreach.

www.parkinson.org
Toll-Free: 800-4PD-INFO (1-800-473-4636)
Email: contact@parkinson.org

<u>*Lewy Body Dementia Association (LBDA)*</u> – LBDA is a 501(c)(3) nonprofit organization dedicated to raising awareness of the Lewy body dementias (LBD), supporting people with LBD, their families and caregivers, and promoting scientific advances. The association's purposes are charitable, educational and scientific.

www.lbda.org
Toll-Free: 800-539-9767

<u>*National Certification Council for Activity Professionals (NCCAP)*</u> – NCCAP is one of the certifying bodies recognized by federal law, and incorporated in many state regulations. NCCAP is the ONLY national organization that exclusively certifies activity professionals who work with the elderly.

www.nccap.org
Phone: 757-552-0653
Email: info@nccap.org

Caregiver Listening Habits

<u>Rate Your Listening Habits</u>: As a listener, how frequently do you engage in the following listening behaviors? Place a check in the appropriate column and complete your score based on the scale at the bottom of the page.

2 = Almost Always   10 = Never

Listening Habit	2	4	6	8	10
Faking attention, pretending to be interested when you're really not					
Being passive, not asking questions or getting clarification when you don't understand					
Listening mainly to what a speaker <u>says</u>, rather than his/her feelings					
Allowing yourself to be easily distracted					
Not being aware of the speaker's facial expressions and nonverbal behavior					
Turning out material that is complex or contrary to your own opinion					
Drawing conclusions, having your mind made up before hearing the speaker's full line of reasoning					
Allowing yourself to wander or daydream					
Feeling restless, impatient or eager to end the conversation					
Interrupting the speaker, taking over the conversation to get to your own side of things					

90-100	Superior Listener
80-89	Very Good Listener
70-79	Good Listener
60-69	Average Listener
50-59	Below Average Listener
0-49	Far Below Average Listener (Pay Attention Today!)

Dementia Behavior Log

Client Name _____

Behavior to be assessed _____

Describe specific client behaviors such as spitting out pills or withdrawing. Avoid general behavioral words such as aggressive, violent or sullen.

Date/Time	Specific Behavior	What happened before? Who was present?	Family/Caregiver Response

Personal History Form

This is _____'s Personal History

Name: _____ Maiden Name: _____

D.O.B.: _____ Preferred Name: _____

Name and relationship of people completing this history:

_____

_____

_____

What age do you think he/she thinks they are? _____

Does he/she ask for their spouse but do not recognize them? _____

Does he/she look for their children but do not recognize them? _____

Does he/she look for their mom? _____

Does he/she perceive themself as younger? Please describe. _____

_____

Describe the "home" he/she remembers. _____

_____

Describe the person's personality prior to onset of disease. _____

_____

What makes the person feel valued? (Talents, occupation, accomplishments, family, etc.)

_____

What are some favorite items they must always have in sight or close by?

_____

What is his/her exact morning routine?

_____

_____

What is his/her exact evening routine?

Type of clothing he/she prefers, and do they like to choose it or have it laid out for them?

What is his/her favorite beverage?

What is his/her favorite food?

What will get him/her motivated? (Church, friends visiting, going out, etc.)

List significant interest in their life: hobbies, recreational, job related, military, etc.

- Age 8 to 20:

- Age 20 to 40:

Religious background? (Affiliation, prayer time, symbols, traditions, church name, etc.)

What type(s) of music does he/she like? Give examples of any musical talents.
_____
_____

What is his/her favorite TV program? Movie?
_____
_____

Can he/she tell the difference between someone on TV and a real person? _____
_____
_____

Marital Status: If married more than once, give specifics. Include names, dates, and relevant information.
_____
_____

List distinct characteristics about spouse. (Occupation, personality or daily routine.)
_____
_____
_____

Does he/she have children? If yes, give names, birth dates, and any relevant information.
_____
_____
_____

Who does he/she ask for the most? What is their relationship? Describe how that person spends his/her day.
_____
_____
_____

What causes stress to him/her?

_____
_____
_____
_____

What calms him/her down when stressed or agitated?

_____
_____
_____
_____

Other information that would help bring joy to your senior:

_____
_____
_____
_____

P = Past interest, **C** = Currently engages in this activity, **NEW** = Has expressed interest in learning

NAME:									
Interest	N/A	P	C	NEW	Interest	N/A	P	C	New
Arts & Crafts					Television / Movies				
Knits					Favorite Channel:				
Sews					Movie Types:				
Crochets					Soap Operas:				
Embroiders					Games Shows:				
Scrapbooks					Talk Shows:				
Paints type:					Comedies:				
Coloring					Dramas:				
Woodworking					News:				
Other					Westerns:				
Table Games					Cartoons:				
Cards type:					Adult Films:				
Bingo					Other:				
Dominoes					Reading / Writing				
Board Games					Book Club				
Pokeno					Type of Books:				
Jigsaw Puzzles:					Large Print				
Other					Talking Books				
Spiritual					Magazines:				
Attend Church					Legacy Kits / Autobiography				
Rosary Service					Newspaper:				
Bible Trivia					Word Search				
Bible Study					Crossword Puzzles				
Reads Bible / Torah / Koran					Letter Writing				
Other:					Other:				

NAME:

Interest	N/A	P	C	NEW	Interest	N/A	P	C	New
Sports Play or watch					**Technology**				
Exercise:					Computers / Internet				
Baseball Team:					Hand-held Video Game:				
Football Team:					TV Video Games:				
Soccer Team:					Other:				
Golf Player:					**Volunteering**				
Basketball Team:					Distribute Mail:				
NASCAR Driver:					Newsletters:				
Tennis Player:					Church Groups:				
Other:					Service Projects:				
Musical Interests					Other:				
Singing					**Social Activities**				
Listening to Radio / CD Type:					Men's Group / Ladies' Group / Young Person's Groups				
Live Music					Happy Hour				
Play Instrument					Coffee Club				
Movies / Videos					Intergenerational Visits				
Outdoor Activities					Discussion Groups				
Gardening					History Groups				
Shopping / Outings					Other:				
Traveling					**Cooking:**				
Hunting					**Animals:**				
Fishing					**Political Interest:**				
Smoking					**Manicures**				

P = Past interest, **C** = Currently engages in this activity, **NEW** = Has expressed interest in learning

Congratulations!

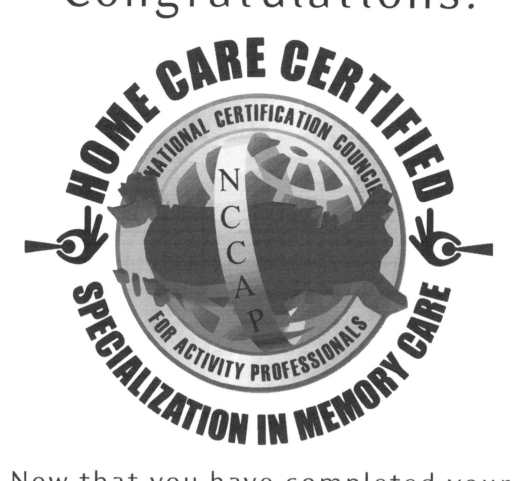

Now that you have completed your Activities 101 Complete course, you are well on your way to Home Care Certification. And, don't forget that you can apply for a specialization in Memory Care with just 10 additional hours of study!

If you have any questions, contact your instructor or call: 888 352-9788

Made in the USA
Lexington, KY
06 July 2016